The Frontier Nurse Practitioner

D0861842

Lynn Jakobs, PhD, FNP-C, is a family nurse practitioner with nearly 20 years of experience practicing in a frontier setting. Dr. Jakobs earned her doctoral degree in nursing at the University of North Dakota, her Master of Science in Nursing at California State University at Sacramento, and her family nurse practitioner certification at the University of California, Davis. She is an instructor at California State University, Fresno, and currently practices at Sierra Family Medical Clinic in North San Juan, a small rural community in northern California. Dr. Jakobs is an avid researcher of rural and frontier nursing and is an active member of the Rural Nurses Organization, the Western Institute of Nursing, and the American Academy of Nurse Practitioners.

The Frontier Nurse Practitioner

A Conceptual Model for Remote-Rural Practice

Lynn Jakobs, PhD, FNP-C

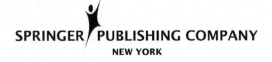

SPRINGER / PUBLISHING COMPANY
NEW YORK

Springer Publishing Company, LLC
11 West 42nd Street
New York, NY 10036
www.springerpub.com

Acquisitions Editor: Suzanne Toppy
Compositor: S4Carlisle Publishing Services

ISBN: 978-0-8261-6911-2
e-book ISBN: 978-0-8261-6912-9

17 18 19 20/5 4 3 2 1

The author and the publisher of this Work have made every effort to use sources believed to be reliable to provide information that is accurate and compatible with the standards generally accepted at the time of publication. Because medical science is continually advancing, our knowledge base continues to expand. Therefore, as new information becomes available, changes in procedures become necessary. We recommend that the reader always consult current research and specific institutional policies before performing any clinical procedure. The author and publisher shall not be liable for any special, consequential, or exemplary damages resulting, in whole or in part, from the readers' use of, or reliance on, the information contained in this book. The publisher has no responsibility for the persistence or accuracy of URLs for external or third-party Internet websites referred to in this publication and does not guarantee that any content on such websites is, or will remain, accurate or appropriate.

Library of Congress Cataloging-in-Publication Data

Names: Jakobs, Lynn, author.
Title: The frontier nurse practitioner : a conceptual model for remote-rural
    practice / Lynn Jakobs.
Description: New York : Springer Publishing Company, [2017] | Includes
    bibliographical references and index.
Identifiers: LCCN 2017004714| ISBN 9780826169112 | ISBN 9780826169129 (e-book)
Subjects: | MESH: Rural Nursing | Nurse Practitioners | Nursing Theory |
    Models, Nursing | United States
Classification: LCC RT82.8 | NLM WY 128 | DDC 610.7306/92--dc23 LC record available at
https://lccn.loc.gov/2017004714

Contact us to receive discount rates on bulk purchases. We can also customize our books to meet your needs. For more information please contact: sales@springerpub.com

Printed in the United States of America by Gasch Printing.

*This book is dedicated to my daughter-in-law,
Karyn Jakobs, who lost her battle with medullary thyroid
cancer shortly after this book was completed.
Her bravery in seeking and undertaking frontier,
or cutting-edge, treatments will hopefully lead
to a cure for this rare cancer.*

Contents

PART III. THE MODEL

Foreword

Nurses have been practicing in remote and rural settings for centuries, yet there remains a paucity of theoretical and conceptual models to explain remote and rural nursing practice. In the 1970s, faculty and graduate students at Montana State University College of Nursing began work to develop a theory base to guide the practice of rural nursing. In the resulting rural nursing theory, rural nurses were described as expert generalists (Long & Weinert, 1989) who must deal with a lack of anonymity and isolation from professional peers. Rural nursing practice was also characterized by role diffusion, as skills were needed to practice in settings that were "a long way from anywhere and pretty close to nowhere" (Scharff, 1998, p. 21). Rural hospital nurses routinely performed a multitude of diverse and unrelated tasks, often during the same shift, and practiced within the realm of other disciplines, including pharmacy, dietary, medicine, social work, and others (Scharff, 1998). Recommendations based on this early work to provide a theoretical foundation for rural nursing practice called for additional rigorous research across diverse settings; over the years, faculty and graduate students have continued to work on the theoretical underpinnings of rural nursing practice (Lee, 1998; Lee & Winters, 2006; Winters, 2013; Winters & Lee, 2010).

A robust theory of rural nursing practice has been hampered by differing definitions of *rural*; problems with conceptual clarity, operationalization, and measurement of rural; and the scarcity of rigorous, large-scale, comparison studies focused on remote and rural nursing practice (Weinert, 2002). One very important area requiring attention is the role of advanced practice nurses in remote and rural settings. Does the description of rural nurses as expert generalists apply to nurse practitioners and nurses in other advanced practice roles? Do advanced practice nurses experience professional isolation, lack anonymity, or do they practice a diverse role that intersects with the roles of other disciplines? What are the barriers to understanding remote and rural advanced nursing practice? Many of these issues are addressed in *The Frontier Nurse Practitioner: A Conceptual Model for Remote-Rural Practice.* Lynn Jakobs contributes to our understanding of remote and rural nursing and provides a strong foundation for additional research into the role of the frontier nurse practitioner. This text makes a significant contribution to our understanding of remote and rural practice and will be of interest to administrators, educators, and clinicians.

Charlene A. Winters, PhD, RN
Professor
Montana State University
College of Nursing
Missoula, Montana

REFERENCES

Lee, H. J. (1998). *Conceptual basis for rural nursing.* New York, NY: Springer Publishing.

Lee, H. J., & Winters, C. A. (Eds.). (2006). *Rural nursing: Concepts, theory, and practice* (2nd ed.). New York, NY: Springer Publishing.

Long, K. A., & Weinert, C. (1989). Rural nursing: Developing the theory base. *Scholarly Inquiry for Nursing Practice, 3*(2), 113–127.

Scharff, J. (1998). The distinctive nature and scope of rural nursing practice: Philosophical bases. In H. J. Lee & C. A. Winters (Eds.), *Rural nursing: Concepts, theory and practice* (2nd ed., pp. 79–196). New York, NY: Springer Publishing.

Weinert, C. (2002). Rural nursing research: Riddle, rhyme, reality. *Communicating Nursing Research, 35,* 37–49.

Winters, C. A. (Ed.). (2013). *Rural nursing: Concepts, theory, and practice* (4th ed.). New York, NY: Springer Publishing.

Winters, C. A., & Lee, H. J. (2010). *Rural nursing: Concepts, theory, and practice* (3rd ed.). New York, NY: Springer Publishing.

Preface

This book is the culmination of nearly 20 years of frontier nurse practitioner (NP) practice and research. It is based on a narrative inquiry study completed in partial fulfillment of a PhD in nursing from the University of North Dakota. The university is located in a frontier state, one with miles of farmlands dotted with small towns—*my kind of place*.

I was raised in a city but moved to the country during high school. Eventually my rural town grew too large and I moved to the frontier. I feel at home and safe in the frontier, a place where people watch out for one another. My youngest child went to high school in a frontier community and I always say that he grew up in "Mayberry." Like the kids in fictional Mayberry, these frontier children didn't have wi-fi or high-speed Internet. The streets were safe and they were free to ride bikes, raft down the river, snow-sled down the hillsides, and just be kids. When the "kids" started their sophomore year in high school, many became cadets in the volunteer fire department. This taught them responsibility and helped shape their values. I hear people say that small-town schools don't have enough to offer young people, but they may not realize that when there are only 60 to 80 students in a K–12 school, you can play varsity basketball even if you're 5′ 5″, you can have a part in the school play even if you can't act, there is a place for everyone on the school council, and home games are the hottest ticket in town. If a student lacks money for a field trip, the entire community pitches in to make sure he or she can go. These facets of small-town life make children, as they grow up, feel protected and valued. This description may represent an idealized version of frontier communities, but it was my experience and the experience of the participants in this book.

I discovered early in my training that frontier NP practice was different from practice in other settings. During classroom discussions with my rural classmates and meetings with my advisor, I began to realize that my frontier practice experiences were uniquely different. I generally saw fewer patients per day and had to manage a wider variety of patient problems with fewer resources. My advisor was continually impressed at the complexity of patient problems that were seen at my clinic site. Even though the NP program had a rural focus, my advisor repeatedly stated how surprised he was at the differences between my clinical site and those of his *rural* students. One particular difference was that my fellow students were not seeing trauma or emergency patients in their family practice clinics. If a patient presented with an unsuspected urgent cardiac issue, an ambulance would be dispatched to handle the problem. When a trauma or emergent cardiac patient presented to my clinic, we would call the volunteer ambulance and manage the patient during transport. Patients were transported to the nearest hospital, 1 hour away, or to the helicopter landing zone 20 minutes from the clinic.

My preceptor and I made house calls, provided hospice care, managed inmate health problems at the county jail, and provided oversight for the local ambulance service. When a flood damaged the highway between two communities on our side of the county, my preceptor and I traveled off-road in a four-wheel drive vehicle to provide health care to an isolated town 20 miles away. We did this weekly until the road was repaired.

I enjoyed the autonomy and variety the clinic provided; therefore, after graduation I accepted a full-time position there. Transitioning from student to the sole health care provider for an entire community was more difficult than I had imagined. This was surprising as I had spent so much clinical time there. We each took call approximately 64 hours per week plus every other weekend and worked 3 regular clinic days per week. Three weeks after graduation, my preceptor, now clinic partner, left for a month-long trip at the height of the tourist season. I found myself wakened during the nights to manage urgent and emergent problems, and then up in the morning to start a full day at the clinic. I was relieved when the clinic hired a *locum tenens* physician to cover weekends while my clinic partner was gone.

Despite the challenges, I truly loved working in a frontier setting. I learned more than I could have imagined from caring for this unique community. Nearly 20 years of experience working in a remote clinic has given me a unique perspective into the rewards and challenges of being a frontier NP. The past experiences with fellow students, my advisor, reading the literature, and, presently, my colleagues, have led me to believe that little is still known about the role and experiences of frontier

NPs. Through the sharing of even short stories of frontier NP experience, problematic situations unique to the frontier setting are brought to light.

It is my hope that the model developed for this book will act as a guide for NPs who wish to venture into the frontier and for the educators who prepare them to do so. The narratives also shed light on federal policies that have shaped and continue to shape frontier health care. Since 2010, 48 rural hospitals have closed and another 283 are on the verge of closing (Gugliotta, 2015). This places the health care of tens of thousands of people in jeopardy. The narratives in this book indicate that frontier clinics are not faring well, either.

The NP role was conceptualized to provide health care to the underserved; frontier communities certainly meet that definition. NPs must not only heed the call to provide services in these communities, they must also advocate for health care equity for frontier dwellers. I hope this book will speak to those NPs who thrive on challenge, desire autonomy, and are not afraid to, as one participant stated, *take the road less traveled.*

Lynn Jakobs

REFERENCE

Gugliotta, G. (2015, March 17). Rural hospital closures increasing. *Daily Yonder.* Retrieved from www.dailyyonder.com/rural-hospitals-face -increasing-pressure/2015/03/17/7771

Acknowledgments

I wish to express my sincere appreciation to the members of my advisory committee for their guidance and support during my time in the doctoral program at the University of North Dakota.

I want to express my appreciation to the participants in this inquiry who gave their time freely and narrated wonderful stories.

I also want to thank the residents of my frontier community. They were not only my patients, but also my friends and neighbors. I am eternally grateful for my frontier journey with them.

I

The Frontier

Part I introduces *the frontier* and the challenges faced by those who live, work, and provide health care in remote areas of the United States. Its purpose is to provide readers with a contextual picture of the environment in which frontier nurse practitioners (NPs) work and the geo-socio-politico-economic forces that influence their practice. This includes definitions, demographics, socioeconomics, workforce issues, and health care systems. The first chapter introduces the concept of frontier and introduces a new federal taxonomy that categorizes U.S. rural and frontier areas by their level of remoteness. Part I also introduces frontier NP practice as a *specialty* practice that requires knowledge, skills, and preparation *different* from those required by NPs working in more populated settings. The last chapter presents practice concepts embedded in the extant literature of both rural and frontier NP practice. These concepts provide the framework for a conceptual model *of* frontier NP practice that is supported by the narrative evidence in Part II of this book.

1

Life in the Frontier

The term *frontier nurse practitioner* (NP) is based on the notion of *place* as central to practice; that place is the frontier. To understand how the frontier impacts nursing practice, one must first understand the nature of life on the frontier. This chapter introduces the concept of frontier and provides definitions and demographic data specific to the concept.

A literature search using the keyword "frontier" brings up articles that involve two conceptualizations of the word. Most utilize the term *frontier* to describe new or cutting-edge research or practice. However, a few articles representing a less abstract meaning of the term frontier are also found. These articles refer to the frontier as a sparsely populated area—a place where either few people have traveled to or where few people live. There is a valid reason for the paucity of articles in the nursing literature that utilize the keyword frontier as a geographic designation: the term is relatively new. Prior to the late 1980s, the government classified very remote or sparsely populated areas as rural. Therefore, the differentiation between rural and frontier is a fairly new phenomenon, and the majority of extant nursing literature does not make this distinction.

The notion of a remote, sparsely populated area is the basis for the concept of frontier as utilized in this book. Frontier lands have been termed *borderlands,* as they lie between the last remnants of civilization and the wilderness. This term could also describe the *place* where frontier NPs practice: the intersection, or borderland, of nursing and medicine.

▪ RURAL AND FRONTIER TAXONOMIES

In 1988, Congress decided that for the purposes of health care policy, frontier is a geographic area with less than seven persons per square mile (Ricketts, Johnson-Webb, & Taylor, 1998). Although widely utilized,

TABLE 1.1   1986 Rural/Frontier Matrix

Parameter	Rural	Frontier
Driving time to next level of care	30 minutes	60 minutes or severe geographic and climatic conditions
Population density	Greater than six but less than 100	Less than six per square mile
Hospital	Small, 25–100 beds, may have swing beds	25 beds or less, or no hospital

Source: Elison (1986, p. 3). Reprinted with permission from Gar Elison.

this definition did not take into account the effect urban areas, which may be located in larger frontier counties, have on aggregate county health data. Over the ensuing years, agencies have utilized multiple methods for determining the criteria for a frontier designation (Hart, 2012).

In the mid-1980s, the Department of Health and Human Services (DHHS) sponsored the formation of the Frontier Health Care Task Force. This group identified specific criteria that defined the differences between frontier and rural health service areas. The resulting matrix, illustrated in Table 1.1, included driving time to next level of care, population density, and level of care at local hospitals.

Despite the 1986 matrix, definitional inconsistencies persisted. In 1997, the Frontier Education Center convened a group of experts to develop a consensus definition. The group identified three key components of the frontier designation: population density, distance, and travel time. The new matrix, Table 1.2, rates each key component and bases the frontier definition on the total score. Based on this matrix, states with the highest number of frontier counties are Colorado, Idaho, Kansas, Minnesota, Montana, Nebraska, North Dakota, New Mexico, Oklahoma, South Dakota, and Texas.

■ THE FRONTIER AND REMOTE METHODOLOGY

The preceding methodologies have utilized county population statistics to delineate frontier areas. This method can be problematic, as larger frontier counties may have one metropolitan area that skews the data for the entire county. In this circumstance, one solution is to designate

TABLE 1.2   1997 Frontier Matrix

	Points
Density—Persons per Square Mile	
0–12	45
12.1–16	30
16.1–20	20
NOTE: Per county or per defined service area with justification	
TOTAL POINTS DENSITY	
Distance—In Miles to Service/Market	
>90	30
61–90	20
30–60	10
NOTE: Starting point must be rational, either a service site or proposed site	
TOTAL POINTS DISTANCE IN MILES	
Travel Time—In Minutes to Service/Market	
>90	30
61–90	20
30–60	10
NOTE: Usual travel time; exceptions must be documented (i.e., weather, geography, seasonal)	
TOTAL POINTS TRAVEL TIME IN MINUTES	
TOTAL POINTS ALL CATEGORIES	

Note: total possible points = 105; minimum points necessary for frontier designation = 55; "extremes" = 55 to 105.

Source: Cromartie (2015).

frontier areas by zip code, as this provides more precise differentiation of rural areas in counties with a mixture of rural and frontier areas (Bigbee, 2007).

In 2012, the Health Resources and Services Administration began accepting comments on a proposed zip code–based methodology for designating U.S. zip code areas as frontier (Health Resources and Services Administration [HRSA], 2012). The resultant frontier and remote (FAR) methodology, summarized in Table 1.3, takes into account both population density and travel time to population centers using a four-level approach.

TABLE 1.3 FAR Criteria

FAR level one	Zip code areas with majority populations living 60 minutes or more from urban areas of 50,000 or more people
FAR level two	Zip code areas with majority populations living 60 minutes or more from urban areas of 50,000 or more people *and* 45 minutes or more from urban areas of 25,000–49,999 people
FAR level three	Zip code areas with majority populations living 60 minutes or more from urban areas of 50,000 or more people; 45 minutes or more from urban areas of 25,000–49,999 people; *and* 30 minutes or more from urban areas of 10,000–24,999 people
FAR level four	Zip code areas with majority populations living 60 minutes or more from urban areas of 50,000 or more people; 45 minutes or more from urban areas of 25,000–49,999 people; 30 minutes or more from urban areas of 10,000–24,999 people; *and* 15 minutes or more from urban areas of 2,500–9,999 people

FAR, frontier and remote.

Source: Health Resources and Services Administration (2012).

(Of note, the FAR taxonomy is one of the few methods that does not rely on a negative definition of rural, i.e., *not* metro.)

The codes are based on urban–rural data from the 2010 census and provide four FAR definition levels ranging from one that is relatively inclusive of rural areas (12.2 million FAR level one residents) to one that is more restrictive (2.3 million FAR level four residents). The original set of codes only considered major road networks in the travel–time calculations; however, the codes are under current revision to include local roads and ferry service (Cromartie, 2015).

The FAR methodology is an effective research tool, as it removes definitional inconsistencies in rural and frontier research. For example, the goal of this book was to elicit narrative evidence from NPs who

TABLE 1.4   U.S. States With the Highest Percentage of Frontier Lands

State	Area in Frontier (Square Miles)	% of Frontier Lands
Alaska	661,306	31.11
Texas	157,786	7.42
Montana	133,133	6.26
New Mexico	108,395	5.10
Arizona	99,399	4.68
Nevada	95,025	4.47
Wyoming	89,750	4.22
Utah	77,053	3.63
Colorado	74,101	3.49
South Dakota	66,233	3.12
Idaho	64,573	3.04
North Dakota	62,427	2.94
Nebraska	57,438	2.70
Minnesota	53,700	2.53
California	52,371	2.46
Oregon	48,089	2.26
Kansas	46,786	2.20
Oklahoma	36,889	1.74
Washington	33,832	1.59

Source: Frontier Education Center (2002).

practice in areas that are remote, where the next level of care may be 1 hour away (see Table 1.3). To this end, participants were recruited from the most remote areas, those which carry an FAR level-four designation.

■ FRONTIER LANDS

The majority of frontier land lies in the western states, stretching from Montana in the north to Texas in the south, and includes up to 45% of the U.S. land mass (Nayar, Yu, & Apenteng, 2013). States with the highest percentages of frontier lands are listed in Table 1.4.

Federal lands comprise approximately 48% of the acreage of the 11 western states, and the majority of frontier land is under federal stewardship (Lorah, 2000). Seventy-seven percent of all nonmetropolitan federal land counties are found in the frontier, and 23% of frontier counties consist largely of only federal land (Frontier Education Center [FEC], 2000).

■ FRONTIER DEMOGRAPHICS

In 2010, more than five and a half million people, nearly 2% of the U.S. population, lived in areas that are considered frontier (FEC, 2000). This number is declining due to population change. This change includes two major components: natural change and net migration (United States Department of Agriculture [USDA], 2015b).

Compared with urban areas, the majority of frontier counties have a higher population of older residents and a lower population of younger adults. People aged 65 and older make up 14.8% of the population in frontier areas, as compared with 12.4% in other parts of the country (FEC, 2003a, b). This high percentage is problematic, as frontier areas are less equipped to provide services and programs to meet the needs of an aging population, such as health care, assisted living, transportation, and so on.

Twenty-one of the 25 counties with the oldest population in the nation are rural. Since 2010, the increase in birth rate (natural change) has not matched the rate of out-migration (USDA, 2015a, b). Although children and youth under age 18 comprise 26.7% of the population in frontier areas, as compared with 25.7% in other areas of the county, youth tend to leave after graduation (FEC, 2003). As residents age in place and ultimately die or leave, the numbers dwindle even more until some frontier towns themselves die. The town of Fossil Oregon, county seat of Wheeler County, is an example of this phenomenon. As one resident stated, "Four deaths a month in a town of 450, the town is just going to die out" (Semuels, 2016). From 2000 to 2013, the median age in Wheeler county rose from 48 to 56, making it the oldest county in Oregon. Due to out-migration of young people, some elementary classes at the local school only have a few students. This decline in student enrollment led the school to start an online distance program to boost enrollment and keep its doors open.

■ SOCIAL CAPITAL

The out-migration of young people can have a negative effect on the social capital in frontier communities. *Social capital* may be defined as the value that social networks and reciprocity bring to communities (Lauder, Reel, Farmer, & Griggs, 2006). Social capital is derived from the notion that social and professional connectedness is at the heart of rural and frontier communities. It is this connectedness that leads to the concept of *close-knit* communities. In the case of Wheeler County, the closure of the only school in town may have negative effects on its institutional social capital. School sports and drama activities garner wide support in small towns. These events cause residents to come together for common causes that benefit the students, such as ticket sales and raffles. The funds raised are used for school programs or after-school activities. In turn, these events foster reciprocity by giving the townspeople entertainment and a sense of purpose and belonging (Woolcock & Narayan, 2000).

Closure of rural and frontier health clinics also negatively impacts the social capital in remote areas. Rural health clinics bring both institutional and human social capital to their communities. Clinics employ townspeople and sometimes serve as the hub of their communities. Health professionals are often community leaders and knowledge brokers who actively participate in the social life of their communities (Schoo, Lawn, & Carson, 2016).

Nurses who work in rural and frontier areas tend to become *embedded* in their communities (Lauder et al., 2006). These nurses contribute not only economically to the community through personal spending and utilization of goods and services, but also socially by volunteering for organizations, working on committees, and sharing their knowledge with others. By sharing their knowledge, nurses have the capacity to increase the knowledge pool in their settings (Prior, Farmer, Godden, & Taylor, 2010).

◼ FRONTIER CULTURE

Culture may be defined as the behaviors and values characteristic of a particular social, ethnic, or age group. Frontier culture is a social culture that stems from geographic isolation. To cope with the challenges inherent in geographic isolation, frontier dwellers often rely on community values, collective coping mechanisms, and social cohesion (Caldwell & Boyd, 2009). The defining attributes of this culture become more evident as isolation increases (Bigbee, 1993). These attributes include a distrust of outsiders, a strong sense of independence and self-reliance, and a preference for interacting with other local residents as opposed to someone from outside the community (Bushy, 2008). This mistrust may have its roots in the long-standing exploitation of natural resources found in frontier areas (Thomas, Lowe, Fulkerson, & Smith, 2011, p. 70). Once these resources were depleted or no longer valued, many of the small towns that supported their extraction were abandoned (Brown & Shafft, 2011, p. 81). This mistrust may make it difficult for outsiders, such as new medical providers, to gain community acceptance.

Hardiness is also part of the frontier culture. This characteristic may stem from a lack of resources making improvisation the norm (Duntze, 2001). Hardiness is associated with self-reliance, the ability or desire to take care of oneself without help from others. This characteristic was observed during the destructive floods in northern California in 1997. Several small towns in the remote Sierra Nevada mountains were cut off from the rest of the state when rivers overflowed and flood waters damaged the only roads in and out of the towns. Rather than wait for help from state agencies, local residents worked together to bag sand from the riverbanks in an effort to stave off the rising waters. When help finally arrived, the locals already had the situation under control. One resident stated, "You do what you have to do to survive, you can't wait for somebody else to come in here and do it for you" (S.F., personal communication, January 1997).

■ SEASONAL POPULATION VARIATIONS IN THE FRONTIER

Seasonal population changes affect the culture of frontier communities via the influx of outsiders. National parks, national forests, national recreation areas, state parks, lands administered by the Bureau of Land Management, and other natural attractions are what draw tourists to frontier counties. These seasonal population fluctuations can overwhelm the limited resources and services in frontier areas. For example, the estimated 3 million visitors each year to Yellowstone National Park create a severe strain on the local health care system in a state of only 493,000 residents where health care provider shortages are significant. In Utah, eight tourism-dependent counties are classified as frontier counties, yet five of these have no hospital (FEC, 2003).

In addition to tourism, there are other reasons for seasonal population changes. These include seasonal tourism workers, *snowbirds* (north-to-south winter migrants), people who own second homes in recreational areas, and agricultural migrants. A report from the state offices of rural health supports these fluctuations. For example, in Skagway,

Alaska, the winter-time population of 800 swells to accommodate 800,000 visitors and 3,000 seasonal workers in summer. Quartzsite, Arizona, a popular destination for snowbirds, can see a nearly tenfold increase in the population of its frontier community in the winter as opposed to summer. In Lake City, Hinsdale County, Colorado, the year-round county population of 760 may quadruple between June and September when summer residents arrive. Most are second home owners or recreational vehicle owners who stay on both public and private lands (FEC, 2003).

A second FEC report highlighted the effects of seasonal population variations and focused attention on the implications for frontier health care systems (FEC, 2006). The study reported that the greatest impact of seasonal populations is on emergency services and related infrastructure.

In frontier recreational areas, clinics deal with an increased number of seasonal injuries such as lacerations, sprains, fractures, and head injuries. These types of injuries test the limits of available emergency medical services that are often provided primarily by volunteers. This concept is exemplified by the following statement, made by one Minnesotan, that "ambulance crews are staffed largely by volunteers" and peak tourism season creates an "unusual burden" (FEC, 2003). In the case of Skagway, Alaska, those in need of emergency hospital services must be airlifted to facilities 1 to 2 hours away. During the summer months, this occurs on average at least once per day.

In addition to lack of emergency services, the lack of retail pharmacies in frontier areas can cause problems for visitors who often either forget to pack their prescription medications or run out during their stay. Local clinic dispensaries have limited drugs on hand and can legally only provide medications to patients who are seen at the clinic for a specific problem. Furthermore, frontier and rural pharmacies are vanishing. A National Rural Health Association policy brief (2003) found that a total of 258 rural communities with a single retail pharmacy in May 2006 had no retail pharmacy in December 2010.

■ POVERTY IN THE FRONTIER

Although seasonal population variations bring challenges to frontier areas, tourism generally improves socioeconomic well-being. A study to assess this phenomenon in 311 rural counties found higher employment growth rates and a higher percentage of working-age residents who were employed (Reeder & Brown, 2005). However, in nonrecreational areas, residents of frontier communities are more likely to be poor. All 50 of the poorest counties in the United States are considered frontier, and at least half of the frontier areas have a poverty rate higher than the national average (FEC, 2003). According to the National Advisory Committee on Rural Health and Human Services, persistent poverty tends to be a rural phenomenon that is tied to physical isolation, exploitation of resources, limited assets, and limited economic opportunities. An overall lack of human and social capital leads to the most remote rural communities dealing with the biggest challenges (Duncan, 2010). Poverty is also regional, as rural poverty is largely concentrated in the south. Those with the most severe poverty are found in historically poor areas of the Southeast, including the Mississippi Delta and Appalachia, as well as on Native American lands (USDA, 2015).

Poverty is closely linked to a lack of health insurance. In 1997 and 1998, the proportion of uninsured was higher among residents of the most rural and the most urban counties than elsewhere in the United States. Nearly 21% of residents aged 65 and younger who lived in the most rural counties reported being uninsured compared with 12% of suburban residents (Eberhardt & Pamuk, 2004). Ricketts (2000) noted that rural residents are more often uninsured compared to urban residents, 18.7% versus 16.3%. In a study on social capital in Utah's rural areas, respondents stated that lack of access to health care or medical insurance was a common experience for low-wage workers. One half of the families interviewed stated that they were uninsured, and the majority of them had accrued debts related to health conditions. Debts accrued because families earned too much to qualify for Medicaid but were unable to afford or had no access to health insurance (Gringeri, 2008).

It may take several years to discover the effect of the Affordable Care Act (ACA) on insurance coverage for frontier dwellers; furthermore, future administrations may repeal or revise provisions of the Act. Frontier residents who are self-employed or earn their living through Internet sales may earn too much to qualify for federal insurance subsidies and, therefore, remain uninsured. While the ACA may eventually be shown to have a positive effect on insurance coverage for frontier dwellers, it may also have a negative effect on access to health care, as many rural hospitals and clinics have closed their doors since its passage (Gugliotta, 2015).

■ RACIAL DIVERSITY IN THE FRONTIER

In regions of the country that have higher percentages of rural non-Whites, the poverty level is higher than the national average (USDA, 2015). However, the majority of frontier counties have a percentage of non-White residents that is well below the national average of 27.6% (United States Census Bureau, 2010). Regional differences in ethnicity exist, with more Hispanics in the southern part of the United States (Rural Health Information Hub, 2010b) and more Native Americans in states with higher percentages of tribal lands such as the Dakotas, Oklahoma, and Alaska (Rural Health Information Hub, 2010a). Less than 2% of the population in rural and small town areas identifies as Native American, but more than half of all Native Americans reside in rural or small town areas (Housing Assistance Council, 2012). In addition, there are clusters of frontier counties in California and Texas that have a higher percentage of Hispanic people than the national average. During the 1990s and the post-2000 periods, the rural Hispanic population grew at the fastest rate of any racial or ethnic group, while the White population grew at the slowest rate (Johnson, 2006).

■ THE FRONTIER ECONOMY

Extractive industries such as mining and timber harvesting have led to a boom–bust economy in some frontier communities. The classic examples of this phenomenon can be found in western states, where many small towns were booming at the height of the gold and silver rush, but went bust when the mining panned out. A more recent example of this phenomenon is found in northwestern North Dakota, in the Bakken Formation, where fracking has led to a modern-day oil boom.

Noonan, North Dakota, is a frontier town located near the U.S.–Canadian border, near drill sites in the Bakken Formation. Its history illustrates the concept of a boom–bust economy. Noonan's first boom came during the railroad expansion in the late 1800s and lasted until the early 1900s, when the nation began to rely on other forms of transportation to move goods. Noonan survived the end of the rail rush due to its proximity to coal mine outcrops. A second, smaller boom fueled by coal mining lasted until the 1930s (Mayda, 2011). In the early 1990s, technological advances and rising oil prices made drilling in the Bakken profitable, and the most recent boom began. However, this boom did not last either, as the drop in oil prices has led to a recent bust in the area. For example, in April 2014, Dickinson, North Dakota, had 203 active drilling rigs. By 2015, this number had dropped to 126 (Reingold, 2015).

In frontier wilderness areas, tourism might be considered a different type of boom–bust economy, as business is said to be *booming* in the tourist season but a bust in the off-season. This phenomenon is seen in Graeagle, California; the town is full of tourists and shop owners in the summer months, but the red-barn-colored shops are boarded up in winter and only a small number of year-round residents can be found. In small, remote towns such as Graeagle, it may cost more money to keep the heat and lights on in the winter than can be earned with the sale of goods or services.

As with Graeagle, most frontier communities are surrounded by public lands. This has a negative effect on the tax base of these frontier areas. The federal government has recognized this and in years past has provided frontier counties with PILT (payment in lieu of taxes) funds to support services in these counties. These PILT funds are primarily utilized to fund firefighting, police protection, construction of public schools and roads, and search-and-rescue operations (Hall, 2013). However, in recent years, PILT payments have fallen below 50%, which can have a crippling effect on local economies (Todorovich & Hagler, 2009).

■ CONCLUSION

Frontier communities are diverse and have characteristics that present unique challenges for nurses—challenges such as poverty, limited resources, isolation, and seasonal population variations. Frontier NPs work in areas of the country that have complex challenges, where emergency services are limited, and the next level of care is at least an hour away. This supports the concept of frontier NP practice as a *high-stakes* practice, owing to the complexity and severity of problems managed by frontier NPs.

Approximately 15% of all NPs practice in rural areas, with only 1.5% in frontier communities (Goolsby, 2005; Kaplan, Skillman, Fordyce, McMenamin, & Doescher, 2012). Although this number is small, their contribution is large. Not only do these NPs support the health care safety net in their frontier communities, oftentimes they *are* the safety net for their communities (Regan, Schempf, Yoon, & Politzer, 2003).

There is a knowledge deficit regarding frontier NP practice. Perhaps this is due to the relatively low percentage of NPs practicing in the frontier, or to the relatively new frontier designation, which distinguishes frontier as a unique subset of rural practice. The lack of published literature and the high-stakes nature of frontier NP practice support the need for a conceptual model for frontier NP practice.

■ QUESTIONS FOR DISCUSSION

- How might isolation and distance affect the delivery and availability of goods and services to frontier areas?
- What types of social capital exist in your town or city and how might this compare to frontier communities?
- If the population in your town increased tenfold as a result of seasonal variations, how would this affect your daily life?
- How does poverty affect the ability of frontier residents to migrate to less rural or urban areas?
- How might frontier and rural areas curb the out-migration of young people?

REFERENCES

Bigbee, J. L. (1993). The uniqueness of rural nursing. *Nursing Clinics of North America, 28*(1), 131–144.

Bigbee, J. L. (2007). The relationship between nurse to population ratio and population density: A pilot study in a rural/frontier state. *Online Journal of Rural Nursing and Health Care, 7*(2), 36–43.

Brown, D. L., & Schafft, K. A. (2011). *Rural people and rural communities in the 21st century.* Maldan, MA: Polity Press.

Bushy, A. (2008). Conducting culturally competent rural nursing research. *Annual Review of Nursing Research, 26*, 221–236.

Caldwell, K., & Boyd, C. P. (2009). Coping and resilience in farming families affected by drought. *Rural and Remote Health, 9*, 1088.

Cromartie, J. (2015, January 27). *Frontier and Remote (FAR) area codes: A preliminary view of upcoming changes.* National Center for Frontier Communities webinar, Economic Research Service, United States Department of Agriculture, Washington, DC.

Duncan, C. (2010). *Poverty and development in rural America's frontier.* Retrieved from http://wwwfrontierus.org/wp-content/uploads/2010/01/Poverty-and-Development-in-Rural-Americas-Frontier_CMDuncan_Feb2011.pdf

Duntze, D. (2001). *The health experiences of individuals living in a rural Alaskan setting* (Master's thesis). Available from ProQuest Dissertation database. Retrieved from https://search.proquest.com/docview/220087481?accountid=40810

Eberhardt, M., & Pamuk, E. (2004). The importance of place of residence: Examining health in rural and nonrural areas. *American Journal of Public Health, 94*(10), 1682–1686.

Elison, G. (1986). Frontier areas: Problems for delivery of health care services. *Rural Health Care, 8*(5), 1–3.

Frontier Education Center. (2002). *2000 update: Frontier counties in the United States.* Retrieved from http://www.Frontierus.org/wp -content/uploads/2000/01/Frontier-Counties-2000update.pdf

Frontier Education Center. (2003a, April). *Frontier youth: Living on the edge.* Retrieved from http://www.Frontierus.org/wp-content/ uploads/2003/01/Frontier-youth-living-on-the-edge.pdf

Frontier Education Center. (2003b, June). *Seasonal population fluctuations in rural and frontier areas: Phase one: The view from state offices of rural health.* Retrieved from http://www.Frontierus.org/wp-content/ uploads/2003/01/Seasonal-pop-fluctuations-Report2003.pdf

Frontier Education Center. (2006). *Impact of seasonal population variations on frontier communities: Maintenance of the healthcare infrastructure.* Retrieved from http://www.Frontierus.org/wp-content/ uploads/2007/01/SeasonalPopVariations-FrontierCommunities2006 .pdf

Goolsby, M. (2005). 2004 AANP National Nurse Practitioner sample survey, Part I: An overview. *Journal of the American Academy of Nurse Practitioners, 17*(9), 337–341. doi:10.1111/j.1745-7599.2005.00060.x

Gringeri, C. (2008). Cashing in on social capital: Subsidizing low-wage work in Utah's rural areas. *Rural Social Work and Community Practice, 13*(1), 20–30.

Gugliotta, G. (2015, March 17). Rural hospitals, one of the cornerstones of smalltown life, facing increasing pressure. *Kaiser Health News.* Retrieved from http://www.khn.org/news/rural-hospitals-one-of-the -cornerstones-of-small-town-life-face-increasing-pressure/

Hall, D. L. (2013, January 4). Payments in lieu of taxes: Congress's flawed solution to the burden of federal land ownership. Retrieved from http://dx.doi.org/10.2139/ssrn.2196683

Hart, G. (2012). *Frontier/Remote, island, and rural literature review.* Grand Forks: Center for Rural Health, University of North Dakota.

Health Resources and Services Administration. (2012). *Methodology for designation of frontier and remote areas.* Retrieved from http://www.gpo .gov/fdsys/pkg/FR-2012-11-05/pdf/2012-26938.pdf

Housing Assistance Council. (2012). *Race & ethnicity in rural America.* Retrieved from http://www.ruralhome.org/storage/research_notes/ rrn-race-and-ethnicity-web.pdf

Johnson, K. (2006). *Demographic trends in rural and small America*. Durham: Carsey Institute, University of New Hampshire.

Kaplan, L., Skillman, S., Fordyce, M., McMenamin, P., & Doescher, M. (2012). Understanding APRN distribution in the United States using NPI data. *Journal for Nurse Practitioners, 8*(8), 626–635.

Lauder, W., Reel, S., Farmer, J., & Griggs, H. (2006). Social capital, rural nursing, and rural nursing theory. *Nursing Inquiry, 13*(1), 73–79.

Lorah, P. (2000). *Population growth, economic security, and cultural change in wilderness counties*. USDA Forest Service Proceedings RMRS-P-Vol-2-2000, Department of Geography, University of St. Thomas, St. Paul, MN.

Mayda, C. (2011). The booms and busts of Noonan, North Dakota. *Focus on Geography, 54*(4), 152–158.

National Rural Health Association. (2003). Health care workforce distribution and shortage issues in rural America. Washington, DC: National Rural Health Association. Retrieved from https://www.ruralhealthweb.org /getattachment/Advocate/Policy-Documents/HealthCareWorkforce-DistributionandShortageJanuary2012.pdf.aspx?lang=en-US

Nayar, P., Yu, F., & Apenteng, B. (2013). Frontier America's health system challenges and population health outcomes. *Journal of Rural Health, 29*(3), 258–265. doi:10.1111/j.1748-0361.2012.00451.x

Prior, M., Farmer, J., Godden, D., & Taylor, J. (2010). More than health: The added value of health services in remote Scotland and Australia. *Health & Place, 16*, 1136–1144.

Reeder, R., & Brown, D. (2005, August). *Recreation, tourism, and rural well-being* (Economic Research Report Number 7). Washington, DC: U.S. Department of Agriculture.

Regan, J., Schempf, A., Yoon, J., & Politzer, R. (2003). The role of federally funded health centers in serving the rural population. *Rural Health Policy, 19*(2), 117–124.

Reingold, J. (2015, March 1). Will America's shale boomtowns bust? A report from the heart of North Dakota's fracking country. *Fortune*. Retrieved from http://www.fortune.com/north-dakota-fracking

Ricketts, T. (2000). The changing nature of rural health care. *Annual Review of Public Health, 21*, 639–657.

Ricketts, T., Johnson-Webb, K., & Taylor, P. (1998). Definitions of rural: A handbook for health policy makers and researchers. Retrieved from http://frontierus.org/definitions-of-rural-a-handbook-for-health -policy-makers-and-researchers

Rural Health Information Hub. (2010a). American Indian and Alaskan Native population for nonmetropolitan counties. Retrieved from

https://www.ruralhealthinfo.org/rural-maps/mapfiles/american
-indian-alaskan-native-population.jpg

Rural Health Information Hub. (2010b). Hispanic/Latino population for
nonmetropolitan counties. Retrieved from https://www.ruralhealthinfo.
org/rural-maps/mapfiles/hispanic-latino-population-nonmetro
-counties.jpg

Schoo, A., Lawn, S., & Carson, D. (2016). Towards equity and sustainabil-
ity of rural and remote health services access: Supporting social capital
and integrated organisational and professional development. *BMC
Health Services Research, 16*(1), 1–5.

Semuels, A. (2016). The graying of rural America. Retrieved from http://
www.theatlantic.com/business/archive/2016/06/the-graying-of
-rural-america/485159

Thomas, A., Lowe, B., Fulkerson, G., & Smith, P. (2011). *Critical rural theory:
Structure, space, culture.* Plymouth, UK: Lexington Books.

Todorovich, P., & Hagler, Y. (2009, March 29–31). *New strategies for regional
economic development.* America 2050 Research Seminar Discussion
Papers and Summary, Healdsburg, CA. Retrieved from http://
frontierus.org/new-strategies-for-regional-economic-development

United States Census Bureau. (2010). Quick facts. Retrieved from http://
www.census.gov/quickfacts/table/PST045215/00

United States Department of Agriculture. (2015a). Geography of poverty.
Retrieved from http://www.ers.usda.gov/topics/rural-economy
-population/rural-poverty-well-being/geography-of-poverty.aspx

United States Department of Agriculture. (2015b). *Rural America at a glance,
2015 edition* (Economic Information Bulletin 145). Washington, DC:
Economic Research Service.

Woolcock, M., & Narayan, D. (2000). Social capital: Implications, development theory, research, and policy. *The World Bank Research Observer,
15*(2), 225–249.

2

Health and Health Care in the Frontier

This chapter establishes the notion that frontier dwellers fare worse than their urban counterparts on many measures of health. Disparate access to medical and dental care, as well as mental health, likely contributes to these health disparities. Public health services are lacking in the frontier, and the majority of emergency services are provided by volunteers. The provision of emergency and trauma care is one of the main differences that sets frontier nurse practitioners (NPs) apart from NPs working in less remote areas. Therefore, special attention is given to the provision of emergency medical services (EMS) in the frontier. The chapter concludes with a discussion of recruitment and retention of health care workers in the frontier.

■ HEALTH STATUS OF FRONTIER DWELLERS

As the frontier designation is fairly new and little is known about the health status of populations living specifically in these areas, rural population health outcomes are included in this section. *Health status* includes data regarding disease prevalence, pathophysiologic process, and morbidity and mortality rates. *Premature mortality*, defined as death before 75 years of age, is greater among rural dwellers than among their urban counterparts. Specific causes that lead to this difference include higher death rates from unintentional injuries, suicide, chronic obstructive pulmonary disease, and diabetes. Specifically, the death rate for persons aged 1 to 24 years was 31% higher in rural versus urban counties (Eberhardt & Pamuk, 2004).

Health outcomes are worse in rural/frontier areas for patients with conditions that account for a large percentage of early deaths, that is, heart disease (Bhuyan, Wang, Opoku, & Lin, 2013; Kulshreshtha, Goyal, Veledar, & Vaccarino, 2014), cancer (Nguyen-Pham, Leung, & McLaughlin, 2014; Singh, 2012; Weaver, Geiger, Lu, & Case, 2013), diabetes (Hale, Bennett, &

Probst, 2010), and chronic obstructive pulmonary disease (Jackson, Coultas, Suzuki, Singh, & Bae, 2013). In rural agricultural areas, farmworkers have a greater exposure to cancer-causing agents, resulting in higher than average rates of brain, stomach, lymphatic, and hematopoietic cancers.

Rural/frontier residents are also less likely to receive preventive health care. From 1998 to 2005, frontier residents had the overall lowest screening rates for colorectal cancer compared to other demographic groups (Cole, Jackson, & Doescher, 2012). In the most isolated rural areas, 78.7% of women travel at least 60 minutes to the nearest hospital offering perinatal services (Rayburn, Richards, & Elwell, 2012) and are significantly less likely to receive counseling related to smoking, alcohol/drug use, and contraception (McCall-Hosenfeld & Weisman, 2011).

Frontier youth have additional risks. Children raised in rural agricultural areas are at higher risk of exposure to pesticides and have higher rates of related illnesses (Ricketts, 2000). Rural counties also report higher rates of childhood obesity, ranging from 17% to 25.9% compared to the national average of 15.8%. One study, which investigated the prevalence and correlation of high body mass index in rural Appalachian children aged 6 to 11 years, found childhood obesity rates of up to 38%, with boys 23% more likely to be overweight (Montgomery-Reagan, Bianco, Heh, Rettos, & Huston, 2009). Teens in the frontier are at a higher risk for suicide than those living in urban areas, with the highest rates occurring in the western frontier states (Frontier Education Center [FEC], 2003). According to the 1999 National Children's Center report on suicide of teens aged 15 to 19 years, the highest rates were in the states of Alaska, Wyoming, Montana, South Dakota, North Dakota, New Mexico, Utah, Arizona, Nevada, Idaho, and Colorado. Communities are trying to combat these high suicide rates by creating strong linkages between schools, health care providers, and mental health programs; however, many of these resources are nonexistent in frontier areas (FEC, 2003).

Frontier dwellers also experience disparities related to emergency and trauma care. Studies have shown that rural areas have proportionately higher mortality rates due to injury, with decreasing population density as the strongest predictor of county-specific trauma death rates (Centers for Disease Control and Prevention [CDC], 2001; Rutledge et al., 1994). Type and severity of injury are among the multiple factors contributing to these high mortality rates, as well as problems accessing appropriate emergency care. Studies have shown that lack of appropriate emergency response is one of the most important factors contributing to increased injury death rates in rural areas (Peek-Asa, Zwerling, & Stallones, 2004); however, studies also indicate that the availability of advanced life support (ALS) prehospital care increases survival rates (Gabella, Hoffman, Marine, & Stallones, 1997; Kearney, Stallones, Swartz, Barker, & Johnson, 1990; Svenson, Spurlock, & Nypaver, 1996; Zwerling et al., 2005).

■ ACCESS TO HEALTH CARE SERVICES

Disparate access to health care has been linked to poor health status. The geographic isolation that characterizes frontier areas poses unique challenges relating to access to, and delivery of, health care services (Ricketts, Johnson-Webb, & Taylor, 1998). The concept of *space*, in relation to space between services and populations, as a causative factor in health care inequity between groups has been termed *spatial inequity* (Thomas, Lowe, Fulkerson, & Smith, 2011, p. 76).

Spatial health care inequity is related to availability of rural hospitals and medical providers. Rural America has 20% of the nation's population but less than 11% of its physicians and less than 16% of its registered nurses (Health Resources and Services Administration [HRSA], 2014). Workforce shortages are especially serious in frontier communities (National Rural Health Association, 2012). Over the past 20 years, the numbers of rural physicians and hospitals have declined due to changes in both reimbursement and rural health policy. Between 1980 and 1998, the total number of community general hospitals decreased by 11.8% due to closures, mergers, and conversions, which in turn forced more physicians out of the rural areas (Ricketts, 2000). In response to rural hospital closures, the Medicare Critical Access Hospital program, part of the Balanced Budget Act of 1997, was developed to financially shore up rural hospitals through the provision of cost-based reimbursement for outpatient, emergency, and limited inpatient services (Reif & Ricketts, 1999).

■ FEDERAL PROGRAMS TO ADDRESS HEALTH DISPARITIES IN THE FRONTIER

Spatial inequity regarding access to health care has been a federal concern since the early 1970s. With the passage of the Medicare Bill in July 1965, the federal government assumed a responsibility for the health care coverage of elderly Americans regardless of geographic residence. Rural underserved Medicare recipients had limited access to health care;

therefore, the Rural Health Clinic Act of 1977 was passed to incentivize rural practice and increase access to care. The Act authorized development of the Rural Health Clinic program that provides enhanced reimbursement rates for Medicare and Medicaid services. The Act also authorized Medicare and Medicaid payments for services provided by NPs and physician assistants (PAs) regardless of physician presence (Wasem, 1990). Furthermore, the Act promoted the use of NPs or PAs by mandating that 50% of the services in rural health clinics be provided by NPs, PAs, or certified nurse-midwives (CNMs).

In rural areas, smaller populations dispersed over wide areas frequently result in economic disincentives for private providers (Wagenfeld, 2000). Therefore, the federal government funded programs to recruit physicians to rural and remote areas. To ameliorate the economic disadvantage of rural physician practice, the National Health Service Corps (NHSC), the largest public program addressing the geographic maldistribution of the U.S. health care workforce, began a medical student loan repayment program to encourage physicians to work in specific underserved sites. In 1991, the NHSC added NPs and CNMs to their student loan repayment program (Earle-Richardson & Earle-Richardson, 1998). To benefit from this program, providers agree to practice in a designated health care professional shortage area for a minimum of 2 years. In 2009, this program was bolstered by the American Recovery and Reinvestment Act, which allotted a $300 million supplement to the NHSC. During the Recovery Act period, March 2009 through February 2011, the increase in numbers of NPs recruited was proportionately higher than all other health care professionals (Pathman & Konrad, 2012).

Federal programs such as the NHSC are limited to areas of the country that are designated health professional shortage areas (HPSAs). This designation is based on an extremely low ratio of patients to available physician providers as well as a number of other extenuating factors such as special populations or geographical distance (Loynd & Constantino, 2008). These areas are further delineated as primary care health professional shortage areas (P-HPSAs), mental health professional shortage areas (M-HPSAs), and dental health professional shortage areas (D-HPSAs).

■ ACCESS TO MENTAL HEALTH IN THE FRONTIER

State and local rural health leaders identify mental health and mental disorders to be the fourth most often identified rural health priority

(Gamm, Hutchison, Dabney, & Dorsey, 2003, p. 165); however, the extent to which the NHSC program addresses physician shortages for mental health care is far less than that for primary health care. This is evidenced by a study of more than 5,000 established P-HPSAs, which found that 29% were eligible for NHSC support compared to 7% of M-HPSAs (Loynd & Constantino, 2008). The extent of this disparity is also borne out in the number of mental health workers in rural areas compared to urban areas. In the period from 2008 to 2010, there were 3.0 rural psychologists versus 6.8 urban psychologists per 10,000 people. In the allied mental health professions, the differences are not as wide. The difference in the number of counselors was 8.4 versus 9.9 per 10,000 and 14.4 versus 17.4 social workers per 10,000 people (HRSA, 2014).

To mitigate these differences, the National Center for Frontier Communities proposes a new type of mental health provider for the frontier, the behavioral health aide (van Hecke, 2012). In this proposal, the locally recruited workers would identify people in need of behavioral health services, connect them to the services and programs for which they are eligible, and help craft and/or implement a mental health care plan. The emphasis on this new type of worker is early intervention and case management. Credentialing and training preparation criteria would be influenced by local needs and vary by state. One of the main functions of the behavioral health aide is to facilitate client entry into eligible programs; however, in the frontier these programs are sparse.

ACCESS TO DENTAL HEALTH IN THE FRONTIER

There are nearly 50 million people living in D-HPSAs nationally, and more than 31 million Americans have no reasonable expectation of finding a dentist in or near their community (PEW Center on the States, 2011). As a result of the geographic maldistribution of dentists, 4,000 areas are federally designated as D-HPSAs, where only 3% of dentists practice (Voinea-Griffin & Solomon, 2016). In American Indian and Alaska Native communities, the dentist-to-population ratio is 1:2,800, nearly twice the national average (American Academy of Pediatrics, 2011). In frontier communities this shortage leads to significant issues regarding access (van Hecke, 2012).

Some states are seeking novel solutions to the problem. For example, Alaska has developed a workforce model that may alleviate the dental care shortage in this frontier state. The following synopsis describes the dental health aide therapist (DHAT) model that is currently in operation:

Alaska's DHAT model is the first in the United States, and is
based on New Zealand's dental nurse model. Alaska's DHATs
practice in remote sites; sites that are managed by tribal
regional health corporations. An essential part of Alaska's
DHAT program is that DHATs are recruited from the rural and
frontier areas where they serve. There are two reasons for this.
First, locally recruited students are more likely to work and
live in these rural and frontier areas on a long-term basis. Most
dentists are recruited and trained outside rural and frontier
areas, and are less likely to choose to practice in remote areas.

Dental therapists are closely tied to their supervising
dentists through telemedicine and phone consultations.
This relationship of the DHATs is designed to be similar to
the supervisory tele-relationships between physician and
physician assistants and includes prospective discussion
of cases, concurrent availability of consultations, and
retrospective quality review of the patients seen by the
DHAT. (Agency for Healthcare Research and Quality, 2012)

In addition to Alaska's DHAT program, another allied dental health
worker, the registered dental hygienist, also shows promise for frontier
areas. Dental hygienists can legally provide direct access care in 36 states
(American Dental Hygienists' Association direct access).

The term *direct access*:

Allows a dental hygienist the right to initiate treatment based
on his or her assessment of a patient's needs without the
specific authorization of a dentist, treat the patient without
the presence of a dentist, and maintain a provider-patient
relationship. (American Dental Hygienists Association, 2004)

Settings for direct access care are often determined by local need,
and each direct access state determines the settings where services may
be provided. These include health departments, community health clinics,
migrant work facilities, medical offices, or offices of NPs, senior centers,
and Native American health centers.

■ PUBLIC HEALTH IN THE FRONTIER

In addition to the lack of medical, dental, and mental health services in
the frontier, there is a lack of public health services. Public health in the

United States arose from the need for proper sanitation and control of communicable diseases. These were largely urban issues, found where people lived close together. In the late 1800s, owing to a more mobile society, urban problems began to spill over into rural areas of the country. Conversely, public health threats such as typhoid, polio, and pellagra were often transported to urban areas through rural routes. The risk of disease transmission and complications of conditions such as hookworm found in rural areas caused the nation to look more closely at rural health risks. A well-known example of early public health nursing is the Frontier Nursing Service, founded in 1925 by Mary Breckinridge. Nurses traveled on horseback to remote areas of Kentucky, delivering babies, providing prenatal care, administering typhoid vaccine, and instructing families on sanitation methods for their homes (Wilson, 1996).

The rural public health movement began with the need to provide these types of services and continued to expand into the mid-1940s when rural residents turned to a newly developed rural hospital system that arose from passage of the Hill-Burton Act (Duffy, 1990). Prior to the passage of this Act, rural residents would have been cared for at home by visiting nurses or doctors. Today, rural public health systems exist primarily to provide services that are population based (Institute of Medicine, 2002). In rural areas they are often tasked with ensuring a clean water supply and cleaning up environmental hazards related to abandoned mining sites (Duffy, 1990).

Although larger local health departments still provide services such as immunizations, family planning, and collection of vital statistics, some frontier communities may be so small that local health departments are nonexistent. In this case, state public health agencies may report only mandated statistics such as overall mortality, morbidity, and sexually transmitted disease rates. In a recent study of population outcomes in 308 U.S. frontier counties, 122 counties had missing data regarding the most basic health outcomes (Jakobs, 2014). Therefore, it is likely that many frontier counties lack the manpower to gather consistent data on population health outcomes.

In some rural areas, hospitals, private practice physicians, and community groups may play a role in providing the needed public health services. However, with the limited resources that characterize frontier communities, there are few agencies to step forward. If a remote community has a rural health clinic, it is likely that the clinic assumes some of the responsibilities that in earlier years would have been the purview of the local health department.

■ EMS IN THE FRONTIER

In 1966, America was in the midst of an injury epidemic. A white paper released by the National Academy of Sciences, National Research Council, titled *Accidental Death and Disability: The Neglected Disease of Modern Society*, found that accidents were the leading cause of death among Americans between the ages of 1 and 37. The paper focused national attention on the regulation, coordination, and standardization of emergency care. In 1972 the national EMS model was officially adopted; by 1978 there were 304 regional EMS systems in operation.

In 1981, the Omnibus Budget Reconciliation Act transferred responsibility for EMS funding to the states through state preventive health and health services block grants. This action provided states with greater local discretion of funding and regulation in their regions. In 2003, a study to assess the support of state EMS agencies in rural areas found substantial variation between states on their approach to EMS issues. It was noted that state EMS agencies focus on regulation and funding of EMS, with only limited attention on provision of rural EMS needs. The study concluded that a new *national* initiative may provide a less fragmented system, particularly in rural areas of the country (Knott, 2003). However, many worry that such an initiative would include a one-size-fits-all proposal for the problem.

Currently, regional EMS systems are physician managed and as such are under the purview of the American Medical Association. EMS providers transport patients to appropriate receiving facilities, which may be a local hospital or a trauma center, depending on the nature of the event. In rural or frontier areas, where EMS personnel consist mainly of volunteers, transportation to local rural clinics (nonemergency facilities) for immediate lifesaving care or stabilization may or may not be sanctioned by EMS agencies.

Within the current EMS provider system there are several responder levels based on skill and training. This range includes: physicians, paramedics, emergency medical technicians (EMTs), and emergency medical responders. The extended response and transport times in frontier areas necessitate basic EMTs having a broader scope of practice than their urban counterparts (Genovesi, Hastings, Edgerton, & Olson, 2014). In remote areas of the country there are EMT-Basics who have received additional training to perform certain lifesaving measures in the field. In some regions this may include inserting peripheral intravenous lines and providing fluids, administering epinephrine by way of an EpiPen, and inserting artificial airways.

Of the five health care access areas mentioned in Rural Healthy People 2010, access to EMS was listed as the highest priority (Gamm et al., 2003, p. 5). This is due in part to several issues: rural EMS agencies exhibit lower staff skill levels, rely more on volunteers, have higher vacancy rates, and have less access to skill maintenance (Patterson, Skillman, & Fordyce, 2015). Although most information regarding EMS is listed as either metro or rural, a recent study discusses the characteristics of EMS in frontier and remote (FAR) areas. Approximately one in 15 EMS responses in the continental United States occur in FAR areas and these responses are more likely to involve ALS as well as on-scene death (Mueller et al., 2016). This is an unfortunate finding as the provision of ALS care in the frontier is made difficult by a lack of ALS-trained responders.

Some frontier EMS situations can be considered *high risk/low volume*, where volunteers are called to life-threatening situations that may only occur a few times a year. In Nebraska, 15% of the EMS departments responded to fewer than 25 calls during 2003, and in Nevada some of the smaller departments respond to between 12 and 30 calls per year (FEC, 2006). Low-volume services need frequent training and practice to maintain a basic skill level; however, higher levels of training are difficult to achieve with insufficient practice. Therefore, frontier EMS are less likely than urban services to have personnel qualified at the ALS or paramedic level. This leads to the *frontier ALS paradox*: fewer hours to train, less-qualified personnel, and a high-risk environment that frequently requires long transport times to a higher level of care (McGinnis, 2004).

Volunteer fire departments account for nearly half the EMS systems in the country (Lindstrom & Losavio, 2004), and in frontier areas, volunteers provide most EMS (FEC, 2006). Due to the voluntary nature of these EMS providers, EMS may be only sporadically available. This issue, along with other challenges of providing rural EMS, increases with the level of remoteness. The National Rural Health Association's *Agenda for the Future* reported that state EMS directors cite ongoing recruitment and retention of personnel as their greatest challenge (McGinnis, 2004). Frontier areas have sparse populations; therefore, there are fewer potential volunteers spread over wide geographic areas. Many remote communities lie in agricultural or mining areas. Workers in these industries may spend long hours on the job and have little time for volunteerism. A North Dakota survey of EMS personnel cited that time commitment was the most significant barrier, not only to recruiting new volunteers, but also to retaining them (FEC, 2006) . In addition, members of volunteer EMS/fire departments are aging, with fewer young people to fill the gap. In rural areas the average age of volunteers tends to be older, with 45% older than 40 years, compared to 34% in urban areas (FEC, 2006).

The challenges to providing adequate EMS care in rural and frontier areas are complex, but the stakes are high. A federal report titled, *Emergency Medical Services in Frontier Areas* (FEC, 2006), acknowledges that not all communities have the ability to support EMS and cites the need for a public EMS safety net. This would require additional grant programs and subsidies to ensure adequate EMS coverage in frontier areas. In 1986, the Frontier Health Care Task Force recommended that frontier areas with populations between 500 and 900 be staffed with a full-time nonphysician provider, or part-time physician, with arrangements for emergency coverage and EMT supervision (Bigbee, 1992); however, this recommendation was not fully implemented.

■ RECRUITMENT AND RETENTION OF FRONTIER HEALTH CARE WORKERS

Strategic workforce planning is hampered by the lack of reliable data on the numbers and types of health professionals currently employed in the frontier. Despite federal incentives to encourage rural NP practice, studies have shown that only a fraction of NPs are practicing in frontier or other underserved areas. Recruitment may be hampered by scope-of-practice variability between states. Regulations that define scope-of-practice limitations vary widely by state. Studies have shown that states with the least restrictive scope of NP practice attract the highest number of NPs (Odell, Kippenbrock, Buron, & Narcisse, 2013; Reagan & Salsberry, 2013).

Both nursing and medical schools have implemented strategies to encourage rural practice for their graduates. One strategy is to place students in rural rotations, with the expectation that some may find they fit this type of practice and choose rural practice sites after graduation (MacRae, van Diepen, & Paterson, 2007). Another strategy is to recruit students from rural areas, and, through distance learning programs, allow those students to advance their education while working with a local preceptor (Meyer et al., 2005; Zukowsky et al., 2011). This strategy may ultimately yield the best results, as nurses tend to cite closeness to family as the main reason to stay in rural areas (Lindsay, 2007; Smith, Edwards, Courtney, & Finlayson, 2001).

CONCLUSION

Frontier dwellers experience disparities in health status and access to primary health care services. Therefore, frontier NPs work with populations that have more complex health needs and fewer resources to draw upon than NPs working in more populated areas. These resources include other providers, such as physicians and NPs, as well as mental health, dental, and public health services. In the United States, 60% of rural areas are designated M-HPSAs, where it may be NPs who identify and treat mental health problems. NPs are hampered in this effort due to the low availability, accessibility, and acceptability of rural behavioral health services.

Residents and visitors in frontier areas also experience more significant adverse outcomes in terms of emergency and trauma care. Despite the critical need for ALS-certified responders, NPs are not recognized as medical providers within the EMS. This may be due to the perception that NPs are not qualified to provide these services. However, registered nurses with specialized training, mobile intensive care nurses (MICNs), can give prehospital orders and direction to EMS personnel within predefined protocols (National Highway Traffic Safety Administration, 2010). The narrative evidence in this book illustrates how effective MICN-certified NPs can be in terms of providing and coordinating frontier emergency care.

Health care workforce maldistribution also leads to health and health care disparities in the frontier. According to the National Rural Health Association, problems with the distribution of medical providers and allied health professionals, as well as recruitment and retention issues in general, are ongoing for rural and frontier areas. Complex situations require comprehensive solutions; such is the case regarding health and health care in the frontier. Frontier NPs are intimately involved in these situations and should be part of the solution.

QUESTIONS FOR DISCUSSION

- In what ways are health status and place of residence related?
- What might be some causes for the higher teen suicide rates in frontier areas?
- Do Americans have a right to accessible health care regardless of the setting?
- The federal government owns the majority of frontier lands surrounding frontier communities, and many frontier residents

work in government industry or industries related to government business. Should federal or state governments be required to provide services in these areas?

- If you are visiting a frontier recreational area and have a traumatic accident, what is your expectation of the type of EMS you would receive?
- Should medical and nursing schools be required to rotate their students through HPSAs?

REFERENCES

Agency for Healthcare Research and Quality. (2012). Dental health aide program improves access to oral health care for rural Alaska native people. *Innovation Profiles*. Retrieved from https://innovations.ahrq .gov/profiles/dental-health-aide-program-improves-access-oral -health-care-rural-alaska-native-people

American Academy of Pediatrics. (2011). Early childhood caries in indigenous communities. *Pediatrics, 127*, 1190–1198.

American Dental Hygienists Association. (2004). Direct access. Retrieved from www.adha.org/direct-access

Bhuyan, S., Wang, Y., Opoku, S., & Lin, G. (2013). Rural–urban differences in acute myocardial infarction mortality: Evidence from Nebraska. *Journal of Cardiovascular Disease Research, 4*, 209–213.

Bigbee, J. L. (1992). Frontier areas: Opportunities for NPs' primary care services. *Nurse Practitioner, 17*(9), 47–57.

Centers for Disease Control and Prevention. (2001). *Health, United States, 2001*. Hyattsville, MD: Author. Retrieved from www.cdc.gov/nchs /data/hus/hus01.pdf

Cole, A., Jackson, J., & Doescher, M. (2012). Urban–rural disparities in colorectal cancer screening: Cross-sectional analysis of 1998–2005 data from the Centers for Disease Control's Behavioral Risk Factor Surveillance Study. *Cancer Medicine, 1*(3), 350–356. doi:10.1002/cam4.40

Duffy, J. (1990). *The sanitarians: A history of American public health*. Urbana: University of Illinois Press.

Earle-Richardson, G., & Earle-Richardson, A. (1998). Commentary from the front lines: Improving the National Health Service Corps' use of medical providers. *Journal of Rural Health, 14*(2), 91–97. doi:10.1111/j.1748-0361.1998.tb00609.x

Eberhardt, M., & Pamuk, E. (2004). The importance of place of residence: Examining health in rural and nonrural areas. *American Journal of Public Health, 94*(10), 1682–1686.

Frontier Education Center. (2003, April). *Frontier youth: Living on the edge.* Retrieved from www.Frontierus.org/wp-content/uploads/2003/01/Frontier-youth-living-on-the-edge.pdf

Frontier Education Center. (2006, April). *Emergency medical services in frontier areas: Volunteer community organizations.* Retrieved from www.Frontierus.org/wp-content/uploads/2006/01/EmergencyMedicalServicesFrontierAreas.pdf

Gabella, B., Hoffman, R., Marine, W., & Stallones, L. (1997). Urban and rural traumatic brain injuries in Colorado. *Annals of Epidemiology, 7,* 207–212.

Gamm, L., Hutchison, L., Dabney, B., & Dorsey, A. (Eds.). (2003). *Rural Healthy People 2010: A companion document to Healthy People 2010, 1.* College Station: The Texas A&M University System Health Science Center, School of Rural Public Health, Southwest Rural Health Research Center.

Genovesi, A., Hastings, B., Edgerton, E., & Olson, L. (2014). Pediatric emergency care capabilities of Indian Health Service emergency medical service agencies serving American Indians/Alaska Natives in rural and frontier areas. *Rural and Remote Health, 14*(2), 2688.

Hale, N., Bennett, K., & Probst, J. (2010). Diabetes care and outcomes: Disparities across rural America. *Journal of Community Health, 35*(4), 365–374. doi:10.1007/s10900-010-9259-0.

Health Resources and Services Administration. (2014). *Distribution of U.S. health care providers residing in rural & urban areas.* Retrieved from https://www.ruralhealthinfo.org/pdf/rural-urban-workforce-distribution-nchwa-2014.pdf

Health Resources and Services Administration. (2014). *Health Workforce analysis.* Retrieved from http://bhpr.hrsa.gov/healthworkforce/index.html

Institute of Medicine. (2002). *The future of the public's health in the 21st century.* Washington, DC: National Academies Press.

Jackson, B., Coultas, D., Suzuki, S., Singh, K., & Bae, S. (2013). Rural–urban disparities in quality of life among patients with COPD. *The Journal of Rural Health, 29*(Suppl. 1), s62–s69. doi:10.1111/jrh.12005

Jakobs, L. (2014, July). *APRNs and the population's health in frontier communities.* Poster presentation at the International Rural Health and Rural Nursing Research Conference, Bozeman, MT.

Kearney, P., Stallones, L., Swartz, C., Barker, D., & Johnson, S. (1990). Unintentional injury death rates in rural Appalachia. *The Journal of Trauma: Injury, Infection, and Critical Care, 30*(12), 1524–1532.

Knott, A. (2003). Emergency medical services in rural areas: The supporting role of state EMS agencies. *The Journal of Rural Health, 19*(4), 492–496. doi:10.1111/j.1748-0361.2003.tb00587.x

Kulshreshtha, A., Goyal, A., Veledar, E., & Vaccarino, V. (2014). Urban–rural differences in coronary heart disease mortality in the United States: 1999–2009. *Public Health Reports, 129*, 19–29.

Lindsay, S. (2007). Gender differences in rural and urban practice location among mid-level health care providers. *Journal of Rural Health, 23*(1), 72–76.

Lindstrom, A., & Losavio, K. (2004). JEMS 2004 Platinum Resource Guide: Need-to-know info at your fingertips. *Journal of Emergency Medical Services, 29*(1), 56–89.

Loynd, C., & Constantino, J. (2008). The National Health Service Corps: Disparities in service to the mentally ill in Missouri and the United States. *Missouri Medicine, 105*(1), 90–92.

MacRae, M., van Diepen, K., & Paterson, M. (2007). Use of clinical placements as a means of recruiting health care students to underserviced areas in Southeastern Ontario: Part 1—Student perspectives. *Australian Journal of Rural Health, 15*(1), 21–28.

McCall-Hosenfeld, J., & Weisman, C. (2011). Receipt of preventive counseling among reproductive-aged women in rural and urban communities. *Rural and Remote Health, 11*(1), 1617.

McGinnis, K. (2004). *Rural and frontier emergency medical services: Agenda for the future.* Kansas City, MO: National Rural Health Association.

Meyer, D., Hamel-Lambert, J., Tice, C., Safran, S., Bolon, D., & Rose-Grippa, K. (2005). Recruiting and retaining mental health professionals to rural communities: An interdisciplinary course in Appalachia. *Journal of Rural Health, 21*(1), 86–91.

Montgomery-Reagan, K., Bianco, M., Heh, V., Rettos, J., & Huston, R. (2009). Prevalence and correlates of high body mass index in rural Appalachian children aged 6–11 years. *Rural and Remote Health, 9*(1), 1–11.

Mueller, L., Donnelly, J., Jacobson, K., Carlson, J., Mann, C., & Wang, H. (2016). National characteristics of emergency medical services in frontier and remote areas. *Prehospital Emergency Care, 20*(2), 191–199.

National Highway Traffic Safety Administration. (2010). *EMS agenda for the future.* Retrieved from www.ems.gov/pdf/2010/EMSAgenda Web_7-06-10.pdf

National Rural Health Association. (2012, January). *Health care workforce distribution and shortage issues in Rural America* (Policy Brief). Retrieved from https://www.ruralhealthweb.org/getattachment/Advocate/Policy-Documents/HealthCareWorkforceDistributionandShortageJanuary2012.pdf.aspx?lang=en-US

Nguyen-Pham, S., Leung, J., & McLaughlin, D. (2014). Disparities in breast cancer stage at diagnosis in urban and rural adult women: A systematic review and meta-analysis. *Annals of Epidemiology, 24*(3), 228–235. doi:10.1016/j.annepidem.2013.12.002

Odell, E., Kippenbrock, T., Buron, W., & Narcisse, M. (2013). Gaps in the primary care of rural and underserved populations: The impact of nurse practitioners in four Mississippi Delta states. *Journal of the American Association of Nurse Practitioners, 25,* 659–666.

Pathman, D., & Konrad, T. (2012). Growth and changes in the National Health Service Corps (NHSC) workforce with the American Recovery and Reinvestment Act. *Journal of the American Board of Family Medicine, 25*(5), 723–733. doi:10.3122/jabfm.2012.05.110261

Patterson, D., Skillman, S., & Fordyce, M. (2015). *Prehospital emergency medical services personnel in rural areas: Results from a survey in nine states.* Seattle: WWAMI Rural Health Research Center, University of Washington.

Peek-Asa, C., Zwerling, C., & Stallones, L. (2004). Acute traumatic injuries in rural populations. *American Journal of Public Health, 94*(10), 1689–1693.

PEW Center on the States. (2011). *Two kinds of dental shortages fuel one major access problem.* Retrieved from www.atsu.edu/mosdoh/about/pdfs/children_dental_shortage_access_brief.pdf

Rayburn, W., Richards, M., & Elwell, E. (2012). Driving times to hospitals with perinatal care in the United States. *Obstetrics & Gynecology, 119*(3), 611–616.

Reagan, P., & Salsberry, P. (2013). The effects of state-level scope-of-practice regulations on the number and growth of nurse practitioners. *Nursing Outlook, 61,* 392–399.

Reif, S., & Ricketts, T. (1999). The Medicare Critical Access Hospital Program: The first year. *Journal of Rural Health, 15*(1), 61–66. doi:10.1111/j.1748-0361.1999.tb00599.x

Ricketts, T. (2000). The changing nature of rural health care. *Annual Review of Public Health, 21,* 639–657.

Ricketts, T., Johnson-Webb, K., & Taylor, P. (1998). *Definitions of rural: A handbook for health policy makers and researchers.* Washington, DC: U.S. Department of Health and Human Services, Federal Office of Rural Health Policy.

Rutledge, R., Fakhry, S., Baker, C., Weaver, N., Ramenofsky, M., Sheldon, G., & Meyer, A. (1994). A population-based study of the association of medical manpower with county trauma death rates in the United States. *Annals of Surgery, 219*(5), 547–567.

Singh, G. (2012). Rural–urban trends and patterns in cervical cancer mortality, incidence, stage, and survival in the United States, 1950–2008. *Journal of Community Health, 37*(1), 217–223. doi:10.1007/s10900-011-9439-6

Smith, S., Edwards, H., Courtney, M., & Finlayson, K. (2001). Factors influencing student nurses in their choice of a rural clinical placement site. *Rural and Remote Health, 1*(89). Retrieved from http://www.rrh.org.au/publishedarticles/article_print_89.pdf

Svenson, J., Spurlock, C., & Nypaver, M. (1996). Factors associated with the higher traumatic death rate among rural children. *Annals of Emergency Medicine, 27*(5), 625–632.

Thomas, A., Lowe, B., Fulkerson, G., & Smith, P. (2011). *Critical rural theory: Structure, space, culture.* Plymouth, UK: Lexington Books.

van Hecke, S. (2012). *Dental therapists: A promising practice for frontier communities.* Silver City, NM: National Center for Frontier Communities.

Voinea-Griffin, A., & Solomon, E. (2016). Dentist shortage: An analysis of dentists, practices, and populations in the underserved areas. *Journal of Public Health Dentistry, 76*(4), 314–319. doi:10.1111/jphd.12157

Wagenfeld, M. (2000). Delivering mental health services to the persistently and seriously mentally ill in frontier areas. *The Journal of Rural Health, 16*(1), 91–96.

Wasem, C. (1990). The Rural Health Clinic Services Act: A sleeping giant of reimbursement. *Journal of the American Academy of Nurse Practitioners, 2*(2), 85–87.

Weaver, K., Geiger, A., Lu, L., & Case, L. (2013). Rural–urban disparities in health status among US cancer survivors. *Cancer, 119*(5), 1050–1057. doi:10.1002/cncr.27840

Wilson, A. (1996). Frontier nursing service: A historical perspective on nurse-managed care. *Journal of Community Health Nursing, 13*(2), 123–127.

Zukowsky, K., Swan, B., Powell, M., Frisby, T., Lauver, L., West, M., & Marsella, A. (2011). Implementing an MSN nursing program at a distance through an urban–rural partnership. *Advances in Neonatal Care, 11*(2), 114–118.

Zwerling, C., Peek-Asa, C., Whitten, P., Choi, S-W., Sprince, N., & Jones, M. (2005). Fatal motor vehicle crashes in rural and urban areas: Decomposing rates into contributing factors. *Injury Prevention, 11*, 24–28.

3

Frontier Nursing in the Literature

It is the premise of this literature review that frontier nursing is a *specialty* practice, one that is on the extreme end of an urban–rural continuum, one that is not well known. The notion of frontier nursing as a specialty practice is supported by Jane Ellis Scharff (2010), who stated:

> Rural nursing practice, be it hospital practice, private practice, or community health practice, is distinctive in its nature and scope from the practice of nursing in urban settings. It is distinctive in its boundaries, intersection, dimension, and even in its core. (p. 269)

If rural nursing is distinctive, frontier nursing must be even more so. Many of the studies and descriptive articles included in this chapter did not articulate the term *frontier*; however, the distinction of frontier nursing reveals itself. Until recently, the term frontier was rarely utilized; frontier research and rural research were simply categorized as rural. To complicate matters further, there have also been definitional inconsistencies of the term *rural* (Bigbee & Lind, 2007). Therefore, as most of the information on frontier nursing is embedded in rural nursing literature, the articles presented in this chapter were ferreted out of searches using the keywords "frontier" and "rural."

A literature search serves to identify key concepts regarding a particular phenomenon. A *concept* can be defined as a complex mental formulation of experience (Chinn & Kramer, 1999, p. 61). Since experience can be collective or individual, concepts can be both public and private. For example, the concept of health has both public and private meanings. From a public standpoint, *health* may be defined as the absence of disease; however, from a private standpoint, it may mean the ability to keep working and providing for one's family. For concepts to be the building blocks of nursing models, they must have public, or professional, meanings (Walker & Avant, 2005, p. 26). This chapter explicates the public concepts related to frontier nurse practitioner (NP) practice.

The studies included in this chapter represent sentinel research that has implications for frontier NP practice. This includes quantifiable information regarding clinical skills and procedures (CSP) utilized in rural and frontier practice, as well as issues surrounding recruitment and retention of frontier NPs. Additionally, studies regarding the transition of urban nurses to rural settings and NPs to frontier practice add rich narrative insight into workforce challenges in rural and frontier areas.

This chapter also includes articles that describe various aspects of frontier NP practice. Stories of NP practice, particularly those told by the NPs themselves, represent significant descriptive evidence regarding frontier NP practice. This anecdotal evidence highlights key concepts related to frontier NP practice.

The information in this chapter is categorically presented in accordance with the major themes found in the literature. Some themes are grouped together, as the concepts and thematic exemplars are interrelated. In addition, as most individual articles include more than one theme, articles may be cited under one or more thematic categories. Many of the concepts identified in the literature support, and were supported by, the theory of rural nursing. Therefore, this chapter begins with a review of this theory.

■ THEORY OF RURAL NURSING

In 1989, Kathleen Ann Long and Clarann Weinert published results from their ethnographic study of rural residents in Montana (Long & Weinert, 1989). The study was based on the assumption that health care needs are different in rural areas than in urban areas. The researchers also made the assumption that all rural areas are viewed as having some common health needs. In addition, the assumption was made that urban models were not appropriate to, or adequate for, meeting the health care needs in rural areas (Winters & Lee, 2010).

The researchers interviewed rural nurses in Montana and identified concepts such as insider–outsider, role diffusion, and lack of anonymity as characteristics of rural nursing practice. Long and Weinert suggested that acceptance as a health care professional is often tied to personal acceptance by the community. Results of their study indicate that community involvement is utilized as a method to overcome this barrier (which may add to the social capital of remote communities).

In addition, they also sampled rural residents in Montana regarding their health beliefs and practices. Although their study participants represented a relatively narrow sample of rural dwellers and nurses, their sentinel research continues to contribute to nursing science and represents the only widely accepted mid-range theory for rural nursing practice (Colledge, 2000; Guadron, 2008; Lauder, Reel, Farmer, & Griggs, 2006; Senn, 2013; Sharp, 2010). Other researchers have replicated Long and Weinert's findings and have identified additional concepts. These concepts are related to role stress and being *on call* as well as issues with confidentiality in small towns (Schmidt, Brandt, & Norris, 1995).

Based on their findings, Long and Weinert developed relational statements regarding health care characteristics of rural residents (Winters & Lee, 2010, p. 10). These statements can be summarized as follows:

1. Rural residents define health primarily as the ability to work or be productive.

2. Rural residents are self-reliant and resist accepting help or services from outsiders.

3. Health care providers in rural areas must deal with a lack of anonymity and much greater role diffusion than providers in urban or suburban settings. In addition, they also reported a greater sense of isolation from professional peers.

In an effort to replicate a portion of Long and Weinert's study and to increase the understanding of frontier residents' perceptions of access to health care, a qualitative study was conducted in a frontier town in southern Montana (Smith, 2008). The specific aims of the study were: (a) to explore frontier residents' health care access to resources; (b) to investigate frontier residents' utilization of health care services; (c) to ascertain reasons frontier residents seek health care; and (d) to explore the residents' overall satisfaction regarding their health care options. Smith interviewed 11 participants who lived in the same frontier town. Ten of the participants described themselves as being healthy; four of these participants further stated that their lifestyle (frontier living and ranching) kept them physically active and led to their feelings of being healthy. All residents interviewed felt they had some form of access to health care resources, even if this meant driving 70 miles to the nearest provider. One participant stated, "You know, we're used to distance, we live with it, it's just a known factor" (p. 44). Three of the participants mentioned informal health care resources, such as soliciting health care advice from a former nurse who worked as an emergency medical technician on the volunteer ambulance or trying to take care of their own ailments using folk remedies. One elder resident stated, "essential oils, things like peppermint; you know if you get a stomach ache. It's like the cold, it's the flu, you know, it's a virus. You're going to get over it. You don't do antibiotics unless you have to" (p. 46). Several participants mentioned the need for local emergency services because "we're so darn far from help" (p. 40). Four of the participants felt an NP would be a benefit to the community, but wondered if there would be enough patients to maintain a practice.

All participants had seen some type of health care provider in the recent past; average length of time from last visit was 1 year. The cost of care was frequently cited as a negative component of accessing care. Patient satisfaction with their health care providers was high even though they traveled many miles to see them and sought care infrequently.

Smith's study provided new insight into the health care perceptions of a small number of frontier residents in a very limited geographic area. Despite this limitation, it validated some of the concepts identified in rural nursing theory, such as placing a high priority on work, self-reliance, and the use of informal health care resources.

■ FRONTIER SKILLSET

A recent study documented the type and number of psychomotor CSP utilized by NPs in the rural state of Oregon (Lausten, 2013). A survey instrument was developed, which included 90 CSP. Among other items, respondents were asked how often each procedure was performed and if they had received training on those procedures during their NP preparation. The survey found significant dichotomies between urban and rural practice. Rural NPs reported the use of a greater number of CSP; furthermore, a majority reported learning most of the CSP outside of their NP educational programs.

In all, 23 of the CSP on the survey were rated by 50% or more of the respondents to be either very important or important to their practice. Results of this survey suggest that NPs planning to practice in rural or frontier areas may need broader exposure to and training in CSP. While the author listed the practice settings (urban, $n = 200$; suburban, $n = 102$; rural, $n = 133$; frontier, $n = 3$) in the respondent demographics, the percentage or number of times the CSP were utilized according to those practice designations was not reported.

In a descriptive article, Mary Ellen Connor (2002) drew upon her varied 20-year career as an NP to provide insight about the skills and personality traits beneficial for providing rural primary care. This insight came as a result of her transitions from frontier to rural to urban practice. Foremost is the possession of a sufficient amount of urgent care experience to handle a wide variety of patient problems. Knowledge of referral specialists is very helpful, particularly when urgent telephone consultations are needed. Delegation skills and familiarity with the scope of practice of those people with whom the NP interfaces are also important. Competence in basic laboratory skills, such as vaginal wet mounts, urinalysis, hematocrit and hemoglobin, rapid Strep screens, urine pregnancy testing, and stool testing for white blood cells, is necessary. Cardiopulmonary resuscitation skills and advanced cardiac life support for both children and adults are vital and must be kept up to date. Good x-ray interpretation skills and familiarity with the radiology group that formally reads films are needed. The NP should know where lab tests are referred and when to expect the results. Lastly, Connor noted that access to Internet resources can be the best way to keep current on research findings and medication updates.

■ EXPERT GENERALIST

The frontier NP has been described as an *expert generalist*, a provider who has training in all aspects of care for all age groups (Rozier, 2000). Roberts, Battaglia, Smithpeter, and Epstein (1999) support this concept and also note that rural and frontier providers often function alone, with few resources and little support. This concept, one of an expert generalist rural NP, revealed itself early in the history of the profession.

Loretta Ford, RN, and Henry Silver, MD, started the first practitioner program at the University of Colorado in 1965 (Edmunds, 2000). Less than 10 years later, Lynne Vigesaa found herself working in the newly developed NP role at a rural clinic in Washington state (Vigesaa, 1974). Vigesaa was a school nurse who moved to a rural area to receive on-the-job training as an NP at a small community clinic. She completed an intense 9-week training program before she and a fellow trainee opened the Darrington Nurse Clinic on April 10, 1972.

The new NPs met with their physician-mentor periodically for review of difficult problems. Their mentor was also available for phone consultation. It was necessary to collaborate with a physician as the NPs found their position with regard to prescription medicines and procedures (suturing, joint injections, and incision and drainage) somewhat tenuous under Washington's new nurse practice act. Vigesaa states that the NPs did everything from attending the delivery of a premature infant to digitalizing an 84-year-old woman. The clinic had regular hours; however, Vigesaa describes her practice as a 24-hour job. The nurses' commitment to providing holistic care to their community is evident in the article. They started parenting classes, a free venereal disease screening clinic, a sex education program, first-aid classes, and group discussions on nutrition, dental care, and alcoholism.

Another example of the expert-generalist concept is provided by Burnett (1999), an NP in rural Idaho, who saw patients of all ages. Children were most commonly seen for upper respiratory complaints or general injuries, with teenagers and middle-aged adults being seen most often for routine physical exams. Elders were often seen for medication management. Burnett cited the organizational skills, solid background in patient assessment, and decision-making abilities developed in the registered nurse role as of paramount importance for preparation of the rural NP. The ability to multitask is also important: she described a scene where she was interrupted while in the middle of an incision and drainage procedure to evaluate, stabilize, and prepare for transfer of a man who walked into the clinic with chest pain.

In rural Idaho, Marie Osborne (Hardesty, 1995) also noted the expert-generalist nature of her practice. She described her practice as diverse: (a) the usual colds, earaches, and pneumonias; (b) the poison ivy and fishhook injuries in the summer; (c) skiing and snowmobiling accidents in the winter; and (d) automobile accidents and falls year-round. She also found it helpful to be comfortable with dermatological conditions, as she saw a number of skin problems in her practice.

Leslie Rozier (2000) also provides a description that illustrates both the expert-generalist characteristic and the multitasking skills required of the rural NP. Rozier describes a situation in which the NP, who is infusing intravenous (IV) fluids into a dehydrated 6-month-old, is called upon to obtain radiographs for and treat an 11-year-old with a fracture/dislocation. The child's family had no insurance, so while monitoring the 6-month-old and the 11-year-old, the NP made phone calls to secure emergency funding to allow the child and his mother to fly to the mainland for surgical care. Just as the NP was accomplishing this task, a resident walked in holding an injured cat, which radiographs confirmed had a fractured pelvis. After giving care instructions for the pet, a call came in: a fisherman had amputated four fingers, and estimated time of arrival to the clinic was 2 hours.

These varied challenges may be the motivation that attracts nurses to rural practice (Mahaffy, 2004). One nurse describes the following scene: The opening ceremony of a new health clinic that community members had struggled to open coincided with both a motor vehicle accident and a bee sting reaction. With competing requirements of stabilizing the trauma victim for ambulance transfer and the need to respond to anaphylactic shock, "we were asking people attending the clinic opening to sit with one patient while we were working on somebody else." Besides emergency, urgent, well, and chronic illness visits, home visits are a routine part of this practice. One nurse noted that during a community outbreak of strep throat, families were sharing personal items and dishes; she educated them and gave each a personal water bottle.

■ TRANSITIONS

Kathryn Rosenthal chose a narrative design to provide rich text for an interpretive phenomenological research study on nursing transitions. The purpose of Rosenthal's (1996) study was to explicate how urban nurses become rural nurses, and through her research provide an educational model to prepare nurse generalists to excel in the rural setting. The specific research aim was to describe the lived experience of rural nurses through their stories. The researcher asked eight generalist nurses who worked in a rural acute care hospital (less than 25 beds located in a mountain setting) to tell the story of how they adapted and excelled in a rural setting after practicing in an urban setting. The author found that four themes emerged from the data:

1. Going With the Flow: Fluid Role

2. Fish Out of Water: Expert to Novice

3. Still Waters Run Deep: Self-Reliance

4. Life in a Fish Bowl: Contextual Knowledge of Patients

The first theme contained subthemes related to role diffusion, a concept noted in rural nursing theory. These subthemes involved the amount of flexibility required by a rural nurse, the lack of ancillary support, and the shifting priorities that faced nurses on a daily basis. The subtheme, fluid role, speaks to the diversity of rural practice and the broad generalist scope of the role in which the rural nurse is expected to function. One participant even relayed a story of helping to x-ray a horse (Rosenthal, 1996).

The second theme contained subthemes related to dualism within the nurse's knowledge base. The participant may have been a surgical nurse, an intensive care unit (ICU) nurse, or a hospice nurse working at an expert level in the urban setting, but now in the rural setting she becomes a novice when working out of her *comfort zone* as a rural generalist must do. Nurses may be called from the delivery room to the emergency room within the same shift or even within the same hour. The researcher states that when urban nurses come to the rural nursing setting feeling confident of their previous knowledge base, their confidence is challenged almost immediately due to the breadth of knowledge needed in the rural setting.

The third theme emerged from subthemes related to the rural nurse's ability to thrive on variety and the ability to stay calm in the middle of chaotic situations. The subtheme self-reliance represents the rural nurses' realization that you are alone in situations, where beforehand, you would have had another professional's guidance or support.

The final theme, life in a fish bowl, illustrates the unique position of the rural nurse where the majority of the patients she cares for will be personally connected to herself, her family, or her friends. Subthemes were identified as: caring for a known person, the discomfort of caring for a friend, the positive aspects of knowing the patient, and how knowing the patient touches your heart and soul. This theme highlights the distinct possibility that the rural nurse may need to care for her own husband, child, mother, or brother in an emergency situation.

Rosenthal's study reinforces concepts that have been previously identified; however, it does so with rich, contextual data that allow the reader to become absorbed in the story and wonder how they would respond in similar situations. This function of narrative storytelling is similar to the concept of *rehearsing for practice* that Benner, Sutphen, Leonard, and Day (2010) describes to promote the use of case studies in the classroom.

Whereas Rosenthal studied the transition of registered nurses to a rural setting, Anna Lythgoe (1999) conducted a phenomenological study of the transition of NPs to practice in a frontier setting. Lythgoe interviewed six NPs providing primary care in frontier settings (operational definition was counties with less than seven persons per square mile), in an undisclosed state in the United States. The purpose of Lythgoe's inquiry was to explore the transition of frontier NPs from prepractice expectations to current practice realities. Participant criteria included at least 3 years of practice as an advanced practice nurse and current practice in a frontier setting. The sample consisted of six family NPs, five female and one male. Four of the six were master's prepared, one had completed a diploma program, and one was a baccalaureate program graduate. Their ages ranged from 39 to 65 years, with five stating they had moved to the frontier area for personal and family reasons.

Lythgoe's (1999) interview guide consisted of four main questions: (a) How do perceptions of the advanced practice role held by NPs in the frontier setting vary from their individual perceptions while aspiring to their current role? (b) What are the successes and the failures that have helped to shape NPs' current perceptions and practices? (c) How adequately do NPs believe they were prepared educationally and experientially to provide primary care in the frontier setting? and (d) How would NPs providing primary care in the frontier setting address the limitations they have experienced if given the opportunity to adjust the preparatory phase of practice? Reporting all responses is beyond the scope of this literature review; however, selected responses may provide insight into some of the concepts that emerged from the narratives in this book.

Regarding the issue of dealing with unexpected complexity of patient problems, one respondent stated, "The role is more complex than I thought it would be . . . there is a lot more to know and there is more responsibility than I really anticipated" (p. 40). Lythgoe (1999) noted a strong thread of independence among the respondents exemplified by these statements: "The degree of autonomy and the level of responsibility are higher than I had anticipated" and "it has increased my responsibility but my freedom has been allowed to blossom" (p. 40).

Working with frontier populations may require knowledge of policy considerations and definitions such as *medically underserved* or *health care professional shortage area* (Hart, 2012). Regarding policy, one respondent stated, "I think the politics are so burdensome, it makes you question what you are doing . . . everything is very complicated and if I could do what I do in a simple way, I would like it . . . but the politics keep it from being simple" (p. 41). Most of the respondents felt successful if their patients had positive outcomes (Lythgoe, 1999). One respondent felt very successful when patients told him that he had made a positive difference in their lives.

Frontier NPs may practice as solo providers who find the boundaries between nursing and medicine blurred. One respondent thought too much time was spent trying to differentiate the boundaries and spending time trying to set and defend them was a waste of time. The majority of respondents felt their preparation was adequate, but suggestions for improvement were to include more 6-week specialty rotations in NP programs and provide more time to practice clinical skills. From an experiential perspective, most felt critical care and emergency room care were the most advantageous prerequisites. Specifically, one respondent stated, "I think we lack emergency care and trauma care in our education. I think we need to be hit hard in the head with emergency. What's the worst case scenario here?" (p. 51).

All respondents in Lythgoe's (1999) study felt successful. They had replaced professional anxiety with knowledge of their resources and how to access answers to their questions. Lythgoe concluded that the successful transition into frontier practice required the development of professional relationships among physicians, other NPs, and other care providers. Four major nursing competencies emerged as Lythgoe analyzed her data: (a) intellectual, (b) technical, (c) interpersonal, and (d) moral.

The strengths of Lythgoe's (1999) study include the rich narrative data gathered. Lythgoe's findings have implications for NP programs as well as policy makers. A limitation of her study is that all respondents practiced in the same state. Although this makes the findings less transferable, the descriptive evidence provides valuable emic information regarding frontier NP practice.

■ PERSONAL AND PROFESSIONAL CHALLENGES

In an article titled "The Advanced Registered Nurse Practitioner in Rural Practice," Schmidt et al. (1995) describe factors that make practicing with rural populations unique. These factors include: (a) creatively addressing the common rural problems directly related to health care, such as limited resources and equipment, and (b) establishing a high degree of positive visibility in the community. They also noted that the ease of accessibility of the rural NP creates a feeling of always being on call. The authors also found that a high level of job stress is produced by treating family and friends as patients.

Other researchers suggest that NPs experience significant difficulties as they care for patients whose illnesses may be beyond their training and expertise and whose suffering is severe. They also suggest that cynicism, isolation, and impairment are potential consequences of rural and frontier practice (Roberts et al., 1999).

Rozier (2000) illustrates the concept of *always on call* in some rural practices. Rozier stated that whenever she took time off to leave the island, where she lived and practiced, the islanders worried about their health and safety; therefore, they would post a lookout to watch for her return. This scenario illustrates the reality of 24-hour call; even though the employment package may call for Monday through Friday, 8 a.m. to 5 p.m., local residents know how to find the only health care provider. Morally and ethically, she could not deny care to her neighbors.

Personal challenges were discussed by other NPs as well and include: (a) long hours, (b) frequent calls, (c) issues with confidentiality, (d) provision of services that may conflict with personal beliefs such as abortion and domestic violence, (e) alternative forms of medical treatment, and (f) maintaining one's professional skills (Burnett, 1999; Dean, 2012; Rozier, 2000).

Seasonal variations in community population can be both a personal and a professional challenge. A seasonal increase of one or 1,000 people does not bring with it an increase in medical providers, just an increase in the workload of the provider on call. Fluctuations in patient population and urgent care issues were just a few of the issues described by Marie Osborne in an article spotlighting her frontier practice in Stanley, Idaho, resident population 100 (Hardesty, 1995). Osborne was the sole health care provider for a clinic that provided both primary care and emergency care for patients, 7 days a week, 24 hours a day. During the winter months, the population increased to 300 due to winter recreational activities and dramatically increased in the summer due to its close proximity to a national recreation area.

Johnson (1996) also discussed these issues. Her clinic's volume and patient population varied seasonally. During the summer 50 to 60 patients were seen a day. Many of these were cannery workers who sustained trauma as a result of their high-risk work environment. In addition to trauma care, this NP's practice included adult primary care, well-child examinations, and prenatal care. She covered the clinic and emergency department every day and was on call every other night, including weekends.

Long work hours are a personal challenge cited by Rozier (2000). In a series of vignettes, she describes challenges particular to her setting. For example, after putting in a 15-hour day, a boating accident victim, a fisherman with a ruptured diaphragm, broken ribs, collapsed lung, and pelvic fractures, was brought to the clinic. It took 18 hours for a storm to quiet long enough to get a helicopter off for the 800-mile journey to the hospital. During the wait, fighting exhaustion, Rozier monitored and stabilized the patient.

The solo NP in a very rural self-managed clinic described challenges that were unique to her setting (Gorek, 2001). Her practice consisted of patients in all age groups. Consistent with other rural and frontier practices, Gorek provided preventative, acute, chronic, and minor emergency care. She also described issues that were unique to her practice setting. These included lack of transportation, lack of specialists, and injured or ill tourists on a seasonal basis. She noted that not having immediate diagnostic services such as labs and x-ray was a challenge in her setting. Mahaffy (2004) also described practice challenges related to the lack of laboratory services. Through community fund-raising efforts, Mahaffy's clinic had purchased the CoaguChek system for monitoring anticoagulant dosing to therapeutic levels and a hemoglobinometer for monitoring patients with anemia.

Role diffusion is another professional challenge. Evidence of role diffusion, a blurred boundary between the role of an NP and the roles of other health care professionals, is present within the descriptive evidence. Vigesaa (1974) discussed how the geographic isolation and lack of comprehensive health services, such as psychiatry and social work, affected the community: "We sometimes must try to fill in for those who otherwise would receive no services at all" (p. 2027). This statement provides evidence of both the role diffusion rural NPs face and anecdotal evidence that the rural NPs' practice may overlap into mental health.

The boundary lines of rural NP practice may also cross over into veterinary medicine. In addition to Burnett's (1999) description of caring for an injured cat, and Rosenthal's (1996) description of x-raying a horse, Johnson (1996) described herself as a "de facto veterinarian" since the veterinarian only came to their isolated Alaskan bush town every 2 or 3 months. In light of this descriptive evidence, frontier NPs should not be surprised to find themselves caring for pets as well as patients.

■ ISOLATION AND EMERGENCY MEDICAL CARE

As noted in the prior section, not every NP may be suited for frontier NP practice. The stories told in this section are from NPs who appear to thrive on it:

> Rural practice can be a lonely, isolated practice. Being rural means turning inward for answers, because there may be nobody to turn to outward. Being a rural nurse means being able to deal with what she or he has got, where she or he is, and being able to live with the consequences. (Scharff, 2010, p. 251)

Bennett's (1981) study adds insight into this concept. Eight rural NPs were either observed or extensively interviewed regarding their practice. Of interest in this book is a quote from one of the NPs who stated:

There have been many practitioners that have come out to an isolated area and months and months go by and they never see their physician. You should search within yourself to see if you really think you feel qualified to be by yourself. If you are going into solo practice, people are going to come to see you, sometimes with acute situations. Your decision is it. Does the person need to go on to the hospital and be admitted to the coronary care unit or can I safely send him home? (p. 120)

Bennett (1981) also described the practice setting of another NP participant and noted there was an emergency room in his rural clinic. The clinic NP stated he was seeing more accidents all the time. Another of Bennett's participants described a situation where a patient showed up at her home in active labor. A fourth participant summed up his response to emergency situations like this, "I felt that there have been some situations that I have been in where I didn't have the knowledge needed to try to make that decision, but on the other hand, I didn't let that patient go anywhere until I had consulted someone" (p. 120). Despite the challenges, independence and autonomy were the most often cited reasons for the respondents to choose rural practice.

The Alaskan bush conjures up pictures of an isolated wilderness. Johnson (1996) described her preparation for her NP role in this setting as a combination of her experiences as an emergency room staff nurse, a paramedic, and a per diem flight nurse on a fixed-wing air ambulance. The medical center in which she and her partner practiced consisted of a two-bed emergency department plus a clinic. An x-ray room, laboratory, and pharmacy were also on site. The nearest hospital was 50 miles away but provided care only to Alaskan Natives. Major trauma patients and all patients requiring hospitalization were treated until their condition stabilized and then were flown to Anchorage, a distance of 290 air miles.

In rural Idaho, Marie Osborne (Hardesty, 1995) provided care for victims of heart attack and stroke, as well as a few emergency labors and deliveries. For the NP interested in rural care, she encouraged experience in emergency medicine, because "trauma care is inevitable" (p. 132). Osborne believed that continuing education programs should be focused toward rural health care practitioners.

Advanced practice nurses working on small, remote Scottish isles describe themselves as being in splendid isolation (Dean, 2012). Dean provides care 24 hours a day for the 150 residents on Eday Island. Prior to accepting a post on the island, she had worked in an intensive care setting and felt prepared to handle trauma and medical emergencies, but required extra training in primary care skills such as chronic disease management. Since accepting the position, she has managed a number of emergency incidents, a fall from a roof, strokes, a suspected heart attack, and a woman who went into early labor. She is primarily responsible for the initial treatment and stabilization of the trauma patients. When the weather is good the helicopter can respond in about 60 to 90 minutes; at other times it can take 6 to 7 hours. The NP works on call 24/7 for 2 weeks, then has 5 or 6 days off. She describes the practice as invigorating because you never know what is going to walk through the door.

Dean (2012) also describes the practice of another NP who works on the remote and rugged western coast of Lewis in the Outer Hebrides along with a general practitioner. Their practice consists of 600 patients and offers emergency visits, childhood and travel vaccines, chronic disease management, cervical cytology, IV antibiotics, and alcohol detox support. Due to a long travel time to the nearest hospital and declining beds in that hospital, she tries to keep patients at home if possible. This includes home visits to administer IV antibiotics to patients with cellulitis to avoid admitting them to the hospital.

Many rural areas have a single economic base such as farming. In these areas, NP practice can cross over into industrial practice and providers need to be familiar with the common types of industrial injuries that they may encounter. At Burnett's clinic in rural Iowa, the local economy is based on agribusiness; therefore, the clinic saw many farm-related injuries. Emergency care was provided for the injuries seen at the clinic, which may be complicated by concomitant conditions such as diabetes. Eyes were a common location for foreign bodies to embed and required prompt intervention no matter what time of day the injury occurred (Burnett, 1999).

◼ RECRUITMENT AND RETENTION

Recruitment and retention of health care professionals is problematic in rural areas and even more so in frontier areas. Professional isolation and lack of anonymity have been cited as causational factors. The outsider status of the professional is also a factor. These issues all lead to difficulties in attracting and retaining health care professionals to rural areas.

Factors related to the recruitment and retention of NPs in rural areas was the subject of a doctoral dissertation (Sharp, 2010). Sharp utilized a focused ethnographic approach to explore the cultural construction of rural NP roles. One of Sharp's assumptions was that NPs experience *transition* to their role as rural NPs and, as a result of that transition, develop a culture different from NPs who practice in urban settings. Twenty-four NPs from across the country with a minimum of 18 months rural practice agreed to participate.

Sharp's analysis focused on the four concepts identified in rural nursing theory: (a) lack of anonymity, (b) outsider versus insider status, (c) self-reliance, and (d) isolation and distance. As a result of the analysis, patterns emerged revealing that NPs who had transitioned to rural practice experienced personal, social, and professional adaptation, leading to role success and gratification. Three of the four concepts from rural nursing theory were also identified during the analysis: (a) lack of anonymity, (b) outsider versus insider status, and (c) self-reliance. The participants spoke about social adaptation in rural communities and were impacted in one of three ways: (a) they either adapted to or accepted a connection to the community, (b) they separated themselves from social situations, or (c) they became part of the community. Those NPs who separated themselves did so due to the perception of potential difficulties with dual roles, that is, having patients as friends. Rural NPs in Sharp's study cited professional gratification along with being close to family as their reasons for staying in a rural setting.

One of the exemplars in Sharp's study supports the concept that frontier NPs are more involved in emergency care situations than their rural or urban counterparts. One participant stated, "We are usually the first stopping place for people that are experiencing emergencies, so you are kind of thrown into probably a larger scope from what we originally thought we would have just because we don't have the resources" (pp. 51–52). Sharp concluded that limited available emergency medical services (EMS) caused many of the NPs to practice to their full scope. Sharp's study is valuable for the resulting insights into rural practice and for the diverse geographic nature of the participants.

Another study attempted to identify personality characteristics that lead to retention of NPs in rural practice. Pat Colledge (2000) conducted a study that evaluated hardiness as a possible predictor of rural NP success. A causal-comparative research design was used to explore the relationship between the location of NP's practice sites and their measured index of hardiness. Colledge defined *rural* as counties with a population of 20,000 or less. Hardiness was measured using the Personal Views Survey, which consists of 50 questions used to measure the traits of control, commitment, and challenge, which have been reliably associated with hardiness. Participants were recruited from Alaska, Washington, Oregon, Idaho, and Montana. Of the 1,148 respondents, 28% practiced in rural locations, with 2.3% listing practice sites in a county that was considered completely rural. Additionally, 39% of the respondents had experience in a rural practice.

A thematic analysis was conducted to evaluate responses to open-ended questions listed on the demographic questionnaire. Nineteen percent of the respondents listed proximity to their home or scenic setting as a reason for the location of their practice site. The least cited reason for location of present employment was economic; however, 19 respondents were practicing in underserved areas as a condition for educational loan repayment.

Reasons for leaving rural practice were described by 28% of respondents and included: (a) family issues, (b) location of practice, (c) to pursue advanced education, and (d) issues related to a rural lifestyle, such as limited cultural opportunities and lack of anonymity. Reasons for considering practice in a rural area were also elicited. Responses included: (a) lifestyle issues such as tranquility, (b) less stress and a perception of fewer societal problems, (c) clinical considerations such as diversity and autonomy, (d) personal reasons such as significant other's occupation and children's educational and social opportunities, and (e) aesthetics of a rural setting, such as the beauty of a pristine mountain community or a small agrarian town. Contrary to results of other studies, only 25 of the 1,148 respondents listed being raised in a rural community as a reason they would consider practice in a rural community (Colledge, 2000).

Colledge (2000) utilized scores on the Personal Views Survey to compute a hardiness index value. Results of the analysis revealed no statistically significant relationship between location of practice and hardiness. There was also no statistically significant difference when each of three traits—challenge, control, and commitment—was analyzed.

Practice locations were then grouped to facilitate the focus of the study and to address the issue of limited respondents in rural locations. These locations were categorized as metropolitan, adjacent to metropolitan, and nonadjacent to metropolitan. This last category represented populations less than 2,500 up to more than 20,000. This category was developed to separate those NPs who live in a metropolitan area but commute to a rural area from NPs who are more likely to live in, and are therefore immersed in, the rural area. The additional analysis revealed a statistically significant difference between the location of practice and a higher score on the challenge subscale of the hardiness index, with the *most* rural respondents scoring higher (Colledge, 2000).

Although Colledge (2000) conducted an extensive analysis of both the qualitative and quantitative data, she did not find a correlation between hardiness and rural practice for NPs. While this study may not have achieved the aim of identifying personality traits that predict rural NP practice, it did provide insightful evidence related to rural NP practice demographics. The respondents were recruited from states that have some of the highest numbers of rural and frontier counties; however, only 28% of the NPs in the sample practiced in rural areas (frontier counties were not specifically mentioned).

Another study found that rural advanced practice registered nurses (APRNs) who feel connected to a supportive network of peers are more likely to continue practicing in rural settings (Conger & Plager, 2008). The notion of professional support and inclusion as conducive to retention was supported by Kanzleiter (2005), who found that physicians and dentists who were included in the decision-making processes of their rural practice organizations were more committed to stay. Kanzleiter also noted that providers' *worldview* influences their philosophy, which in turn directs their approach to practice and their willingness to remain practicing in rural underserved areas. This suggests that the life experiences associated with family and community are more influential in shaping commitment and are predictive of length of stay than mere exposure to a rural practice setting.

■ SUMMARY OF THE LITERATURE

The majority of information regarding frontier NP practice is embedded in rural nursing literature. Although there is descriptive evidence regarding the type of procedures used in rural/frontier practice, Lausten (2013) provides the only quantitative study of procedures performed by NPs in a rural state. Owing to the small number of frontier NPs, both in Lausten's study and nationwide, a survey of this type would likely involve a sample size too small for generalizability. However, both Lausten's quantitative study and Rosenthal's qualitative study provide valuable insight into the broad skillset required to practice in the frontier.

Descriptive evidence regarding frontier NP practice is obtained through individual NP stories. Recurring themes identified in the literature

TABLE 3.1 Summary of Literature

Theme	Author
Expert generalist and multitasking	Hardesty (1995), Rosenthal (1996), Burnett (1999), Roberts et al. (1999), Rozier (2000), Mahaffy (2004), Sharp (2010)
Personal challenges	Vigesaa (1974), Hardesty (1995), Schmidt et al. (1995), Johnson (1996), Burnett (1999), Roberts et al. (1999), Rozier (2000), Gorek (2001), Mahaffy (2004), Dean (2012)
Rural competencies	Lythgoe (1999), Connor (2002)
Isolation/emergency care	Hardesty (1995), Johnson (1996), Burnett (1999), Mahaffy (2004), Dean (2012)
Ethics	Long and Weinert (1989), Rozier (2000)

are summarized in Table 3.1. These descriptions of frontier NP practice illustrate the expert-generalist qualifications necessary to effectively work in these remote settings, that is, skills in preventative, acute, chronic, and emergency care with all age groups. Competencies in radiology, prenatal care, and emergency care were frequently mentioned as necessary for frontier practice. Challenges in this practice setting included isolation, frequent call, and limited resources. As sole providers, frontier NPs must possess the ability to triage, multitask, and use resources effectively. Many authors also noted seasonal population fluctuations, which may increase the number of urgent or emergency patients and add to the on-call stress of frontier NPs. Positive attributes of frontier practice included the wide variety of patient problems encountered (Dean, 2012; Mahaffy, 2004; Rosenthal, 1996), which invigorated NPs' practice, as well as autonomy and increased responsibility (Burnett, 1999).

There are ethical issues confronting frontier NPs, almost daily. Many are issues that NPs working in urban or metropolitan areas may never face. Given the nature of small towns, Long and Weinert (1989) discuss issues with confidentiality, Rozier (2000) speaks to the ethics and morals of being on call, and Lythgoe (1999) includes morality as one of the competencies rural nurses should have. Jane Scharff (2010) adds to the ethical discussion when she states:

> Being rural means that when a nurse walks into the emergency room, it may be her or his spouse or child who needs a nurse,

and at that moment, being a nurse takes priority over being anyone else. Since you are the highest trained and educated healthcare personnel available, you must maintain an objective stance, if you are to manage the situation. (p. 251)

In addition to these themes, the following assumptions regarding frontier NP practice are drawn from the literature review:

- The frontier NP must be an expert generalist capable of multi-tasking and effectively utilizing available resources.

- The frontier NP must be comfortable with dermatology, must have x-ray skills, and may be called upon to treat animals.

- The frontier NP must be comfortable with behavioral health and medications for treatment of depression and substance abuse.

- The frontier NP must possess emergency care skills and competencies

- The frontier NP struggles with ethical considerations when caring for family and friends.

- The frontier NP assumes a heavy on-call schedule and most often works in isolation from other providers.

- NPs who wish to venture into the frontier must value a challenge, thrive on diversity, and use available resources wisely and creatively.

■ DISCUSSION

A literature review identifies key concepts and research findings; a literature review also identifies gaps in the existing literature. Studies have shown that NPs are more likely than physicians to practice in frontier areas (DesRoches et al., 2013; Goolsby, 2011); however, the literature search indicates that evidence regarding NP practice that is specifically identified as frontier practice is lacking in the literature.

The evidence found in the literature review provides powerful, although scant, information regarding ethical considerations of frontier practice such as the following: How do frontier NPs manage the dual relationships that exist when it becomes necessary to have family and friends as patients, and how do frontier NPs promote patient autonomy and protect patient privacy?

Professionals bring human social capital to frontier communities. Evidence regarding the social capital that frontier NPs may bring to their communities is also lacking. In addition to medical care, what other benefits do frontier communities receive from the presence of NPs? To what extent do NPs use knowledge of policy and politics to ameliorate the disparities in health and health care in frontier communities?

The literature supports the notion that frontier NPs provide emergency care. There is a gap in the literature regarding the way in which frontier NPs integrate with local EMS systems. There is also a gap in the literature regarding prerequisite education and training in emergency and wilderness care. What responsibility do educational programs have to provide necessary skills to NP graduates who wish to heed the call of the National Health Service Corps (NHSC) and practice in frontier areas?

The answers to these questions will likely be found not in statistical charts or graphs but in narrative stories of nursing experience. Narratives are an important source of nursing knowledge, as they allow for recognition of both the mundane and the extraordinary in everyday nursing situations (Wolf & Langner, 2000). The knowledge embedded in nursing narratives grounds the ontology of nursing, what it *is* to be a nurse, in nursing experience (Nairn, 2004).

Nurses share narratives in everyday practice. These narratives may take the form of explanations or descriptions; they may answer questions regarding the what, how, or why of practice situations. Narratives may be oral, digital, or written. Written narratives may be found in nursing journals under the title *Clinical Pearls* or *Practice Tips*. When shared with others, narratives disseminate nursing knowledge.

Narratives are situational or contextual. The concepts summarized in Table 3.1 are supported by the knowledge embedded in rural and frontier nursing stories. These concepts are not meant to represent practice characteristics in other settings. The narratives in this book are also contextual; they represent practice in the context of a frontier setting.

■ CONCLUSION

The literature review supports the concept of frontier NP practice as a *specialty* practice—one that has not been fully explored in the literature.

Frontier communities face many challenges; the interconnectedness of the geo-socio-politico-economic forces that shape the relationship between frontier communities and the health care system is complex and contextually unique. This also holds true for frontier NPs and the communities in which they practice and live. Their stories are explored in Part II of this book.

■ QUESTIONS FOR DISCUSSION

- How does evidence in the literature support the distinctive nature of frontier NP practice?
- How might NP students get exposure to the wide variety of procedures utilized in frontier practice?
- What are some of the educational options schools can utilize to prepare NPs to provide emergency care in the frontier?
- What methods might be employed to manage the personal and professional challenges of frontier NP practice?

REFERENCES

Benner, P., Sutphen, M., Leonard, V., & Day, L. (2010). *Educating nurses: A call for radical transformation.* San Francisco, CA: Jossey-Bass.

Bennett, M. (1981). *The rural family nurse practitioner: The quest for a role identity* (Doctoral dissertation). Available from ProQuest Dissertaton database. (UMI No. 303146652)

Bigbee, J. L., & Lind, B. (2007). Methodological challenges in rural and frontier nursing research. *Applied Nursing Research, 20,* 104–106.

Burnett, B. (1999). Rural family practice and the nurse practitioner. *Imprint, 46*(4), 83–84.

Chinn, P. L., & Kramer, M. K. (1999). *Theory and nursing: Integrated knowledge development* (5th ed.). St. Louis, MO: Mosby.

Colledge, P. (2000). *Hardiness as a predictor of nurse practitioners in rural practice* (Doctoral dissertation). Available from ProQuest Dissertation database. (UMI No. 304627597)

Conger, M., & Plager, K. (2008). Advanced nursing practice in rural areas: Connectedness versus disconnectedness. *Online Journal of Rural Nursing and Health Care, 8*(1), 24–38.

Connor, M. (2002). Transitioning to rural primary care. *Advance for Nurse Practitioners, 10*(6), 83–84.

Dean, E. (2012). In splendid isolation. *Nursing Standard, 26*(46), 18–20.

DesRoches, C., Gaudet, J., Perloff, J., Donelan, K., Iezzoni, L., & Buerhaus, P. (2013). Using Medicare data to assess nurse practitioner–provided care. *Nursing Outlook, 61*(6), 400–407. doi:10.1016/j.outlook.2013.05.005

Edmunds, M. (2000). Nurse practitioners: Remembering the past, planning the future. Retrieved from http://www.medscape.com/viewarticle /408388

Goolsby, M. (2011). 2009–2010 AANP national nurse practitioner sample survey: An overview. *Journal of the American Academy of Nurse Practitioners, 23*(5), 266–268. doi:10.1111/j.1745-7599.2011.00611.x

Gorek, B. (2001). Nurse practitioners in rural settings. *Geriatric Nursing, 22*(5), 263–264.

Guadron, M. (2008). *Identification of patterns of knowing used by rural community health nurses in decision-making* (Doctoral dissertation). Available from ProQuest Dissertation database. (UMI No. 304157862)

Hardesty, M. (1995). Marie Osborn: Rural health care nurse practitioner. *Nurse Practitioner Forum, 6*(3), 131–132.

Hart, G. (2012). *Frontier/Remote, island, and rural literature review* (pp. 1–37). Grand Forks: Center for Rural Health, University of North Dakota.

Johnson, E. (1996). A nurse practitioner's experience in bush Alaska. *Journal of Emergency Nursing, 22*, 509–510.

Kanzleiter, L. J. (2005). *Emergence of commitment to practice in a rural medically underserved community* (Doctoral dissertation). Available from ProQuest Dissertation database. (UMI No. 3187522)

Lauder, W., Reel, S., Farmer, J., & Griggs, H. (2006). Social capital, rural nursing and rural nursing theory. *Nursing Inquiry, 13*(1), 73–79.

Lausten, G. (2013). What do nurse practitioners do? Analysis of a skills survey of nurse practitioners. *Journal of the American Association of Nurse Practitioners, 25*, 32–41.

Long, K., & Weinert, C. (1989). Rural nursing: Developing the theory base. *Scholarly Inquiry for Nursing Practice: An International Journal, 3*, 113–127.

Lythgoe, A. (1999). *Transitions: The nurse practitioner as primary care provider in the frontier setting* (Master's thesis). Available from ProQuest Dissertation database. (UMI No. 304556127)

Mahaffy, C. (2004). Varied challenge: That's the spice attracting RNs to rural nursing. *Alberta RN, 60*(6), 22–23.

Nairn, S. (2004). Emergency care and narrative knowledge. *Journal of Advanced Nursing, 48*(1), 59–67.

Roberts, L., Battaglia, J., Smithpeter, M., & Epstein, R. (1999). An office on Main Street: Health care dilemmas in small communities. *Hastings Center Report, 29*(4), 28–37.

Rosenthal, K. (1996). *Rural nursing: An exploratory narrative description* (Doctoral dissertation). Available from ProQuest Dissertation database. (UMI No. 304379526)

Rozier, L. (2000). The rural nurse practitioner. In J. Hickey, R. Ouimette, & S. Venegoni (Eds.), *Advanced practice nursing: Changing roles and clinical applications* (2nd ed., pp. 421-427). Baltimore, MD: Lippincott Williams & Wilkins.

Scharff, J. (2010). The distinctive nature and scope of rural nursing practice: Philosophical bases. In C. Winters & H. Lee (Eds.), *Rural nursing: Concepts, theory, and practice* (3rd ed., pp. 249–268). New York, NY: Springer Publishing.

Schmidt, L., Brandt, J., & Norris, K. (1995). The advanced registered nurse practitioner in rural practice. *Kansas Nurse, 70*(9), 1–2.

Senn, J. (2013). Peplau's theory of interpersonal relations: Application in emergency and rural nursing. *Nursing Science Quarterly, 26*(1), 31–35. doi:10.1177/0894318412466744

Sharp, D. (2010). *Factors related to the recruitment and retention of nurse practitioners in rural areas* (Doctoral dissertation). Available from ProQuest Dissertation database. (UMI No. 3409167)

Smith, R. (2008). *Frontier residents' perceptions of health care access* (Unpublished master's thesis). Montana State University, Bozeman, MT. Retrieved from http://scholarworks.montana.edu/xmlui/bitstream/handle/1/2308/smithr0508.pdf?sequence=1

Vigesaa, L. (1974). The nursing story. *The American Journal of Nursing, 74*(11), 2026–2027. doi:10.2307/3423206

Walker, L. O., & Avant, K. C. (2005). *Strategies for theory construction in nursing* (4th ed.). Upper Saddle River, NJ: Prentice Hall.

Winters, C., & Lee, H. (Eds.). (2010). *Rural nursing: Concepts, theory, and practice* (3rd ed.). New York, NY: Springer Publishing.

Wolf, Z. R., & Langner, S. R. (2000). The meaning of nursing practice in the stories and poems of nurses working in hospitals: A phenomenological study. *International Journal for Human Caring, 4*, 7–17.

II

The Narratives

The narratives presented in this book depict frontier nurse practitioner (NP) practice at a certain moment in time, a written snapshot. While some of the NPs may reflect on their experiences *over time*, their perspective, or viewing lens, is influenced by recent and current events. Over time, governments shift funding priorities. This is certainly evident with the passage of the Affordable Care Act. The effects of federal and state policy in the arena of frontier health care become visible as the participants tell their stories.

Five female and two male NPs narrated stories of frontier practice for this book. All participants were older than 50 years. Bob has 38 years of experience as a frontier NP, Ann has more than 20 years of frontier nursing experience, Jim has 3 years of frontier NP experience, Pam has 15 years of frontier nursing experience, Sue has more than 20 years of frontier nursing experience, Amy has nearly 10 years of frontier NP experience, and Lori has 17 years of frontier NP experience. All participants were initially master's prepared; Ann and Lori have completed doctoral degrees in nursing, and Bob has earned a doctorate degree in a related discipline. All participants are married and six have adult children who were raised in their frontier community.

Bob, Lori, Ann, and Amy practice at a community clinic. Jim practices in a small community clinic associated with a critical access hospital, Pam practices in a private clinic owned by a physician, and Sue practices in a private clinic that had been recently purchased by a large health care organization. All participants are family NPs who provide primary care services to patients of all ages.

Before entering frontier NP practice, Jim and Bob had worked as flight nurses and had extensive trauma and emergency medical experience. Amy had worked as a nurse anesthetist and had intensive care experience.

Lori worked on an acute medical–surgical unit in a rural hospital and had 3 months of part-time experience in a rural emergency department. Sue and Pam had worked in acute emergency departments. Ann began her career as a public health nurse who saw a need for emergency medical technicians (EMTs) in the community and started a certification program. Ann is also a member of the local volunteer fire department and utilized her EMT skills in this manner.

The seven participants in this study represent frontier communities in five midwestern and western states. Their practice settings reflect the geographic and economic diversity of frontier communities. Three of the practice settings are in mountainous regions accessible by winding canyon roads. The local economies of these communities are currently driven by tourism. This was not always the case. Historically they were driven by extractive industries, such as logging and mining, which were eventually closed down as a result of environmental concerns and economic downturns. Two other communities are surrounded by high-elevation plains and grasslands that support an agriculture-based economy. Another community is located in a high-elevation valley and is supported by an agricultural and ranching-based economy. Despite their diversity, these communities share common features such as sparse populations, extreme weather, a lack of general services, and long driving distances to urban areas.

In the following chapters, each participant's story is presented in case study format. The cases are structured in the following manner:

1. Overview of each participant's practice and the motivation for frontier practice

2. Concepts found in the extant literature and concepts that emerged from the narratives

3. Narrative themes that exemplify some or all of the concepts

4

Bob: An Early Pioneer

■ OVERVIEW

Bob is interviewed in his home and reflects on a long and satisfying career as a frontier nurse practitioner (NP). He is considered a frontier pioneer as he created a clinic and a practice nearly from scratch at a time in our recent history when many people "did not know what an NP was." Bob was drawn to the frontier because of the independence it offered:

> I had been a medic in the Air Force and a lot of that training is focused on independence. I would work in clinics in remote areas, for example, Thailand. I would function on airplanes independently, in Turkey independently, and in Alaska independently. This independence meant that you would have medical support but it was not direct, and so you were making some fairly heavy decisions, some fairly complex medical decision making, without the usual kind of institutional support. And so that kind of prepared me for wanting to function in a more independent way.

Bob's story is given particular attention as it represents an oral history of the development of frontier NP practice. Bob's story also provides an example of how federal policy influences frontier health care.

Bob, recently semiretired, began his frontier NP practice 38 years ago as a member of the National Health Service Corps when he accepted an assignment at a newly formed community clinic. Prior to his arrival the community had been served by rotating physicians who visited once or twice a week. The county owned a small house and allocated the main floor for use as a medical clinic. The rental fee was one dollar per year. The visiting physicians had created charts for the patients who were seen at the clinic, but other than a few charts, a small microscope, a donated x-ray machine, and some floor space, there was little infrastructure in place.

The lack of a fully equipped medical clinic wasn't the only issue. "The Corps wasn't real clear on what NPs could do independently in a community," and Bob's new state didn't know what to do with him either, as there was no reciprocity for NPs. He was the first NP educated in another state to apply for licensure. The Corps had a contract with an NP program in Bob's new state and after passing an oral/written/practical test Bob was granted an interim permit (which eventually led to licensure). In 1976, the state required NPs to have physician oversight: "it wasn't a formal licensing kind of thing, you just had to say that you were working with a physician," so the doctors who had previously been practicing in the community on a part-time basis agreed to "provide that coverage."

Although Bob's salary was paid by the Corps, the clinic needed revenue to pay for overhead and purchase equipment and supplies:

> In 1976, Medicare did not pay for NP services. That was not approved. But, there was a program called the Physician Extender Project which was administered through the university system and you could enroll in that program.

The purpose of the Project was to gather data for the federal government to determine if paying for services provided by NPs was a useful and cost-effective way of providing care:

> When the Project ended the federal government approved the Rural Health Clinic Act which then set up rural health clinics [RHC], for which we applied. By virtue of that designation, Medicare was required to pay you [an NP]. Next came Federally Qualified Health Centers [FQHC] which gave you access to a higher reimbursement rate that was cost-based. They would pay you $100 a visit no matter whether it was a blood pressure check or you did a major laceration. Then at the end of that year there was reconciliation of what the cost of the care was to provide it and the revenue that you generated.

As clinic administrator, funding health care for the community clinic meant bridging the gap between insurance revenue and clinic costs. Over the years, Bob found that revenue from grant funding and federal programs changes in response to changes in federal policies and priorities. Bob states:

> There was a shift in funding priorities between passages of the Rural Health Clinic Act in 1977, which allocated federal subsidies based on geographic criteria, and the development of the FQHC program started in early 1990s, which allocated federal subsidies on geographic and/or medically underserved criteria. FQHCs located in populated areas that were considered medically underserved would compete directly with rural clinics for funding. This was the beginning of the movement to shift funding priorities away from geographically isolated clinics to population-based health care organizations.

Eight years ago grant funding dwindled; however, in 2007 the clinic was designated a Health Resources and Services Administration 330 clinic. This changed the clinic's designation to an FQHC, which is mandated to offer a full array of health services:

> For many years about 70% of our revenue was from the patients' medical insurance and only about 30% of our funding was grant revenue. Our grant revenue sustained our 24/7 coverage to which I was committed to and so I went after money to try and support that, whether it was from foundations to buy x-ray equipment or whatever, all of those were pieces of an overall administration of frontier practice, to try and sustain it. Finally they pulled these revenue streams and we were desperate and literally we were down to our last dollar when I wrote that grant for the 330.

While Bob states that the 330 designation was a "godsend," it has also been somewhat of a curse. To maintain the 330 designation a clinic must increase new patient visits by approximately 1,000 over the 3-year funding period. This is not possible in a frontier area where there may not be 1,000 people in the entire county. Therefore, Bob's clinic merged with a large rural clinic in order to meet the requirement for new patient visits (the merged clinics were able to combine patient numbers). To help cut costs, Bob relinquished the administrator role in an effort to sustain health care in his frontier community and within a year he retired. Due to cost containment efforts, the new administration has cut the clinic down to 4 days a week and also ceased 24/7 medical coverage for the community.

■ CONCEPTS

Bob's story reveals new concepts and provides descriptive evidence that supports concepts summarized in the literature review. Stories, or story segments, may contain one or more concepts. In this first story the concepts of insider–outsider, emergency care provider, and personal challenges become evident.

Bob narrates this story regarding his first day of frontier practice in a new community. He feels this experience helped his outsider image with the townspeople:

> We got in late in the evening and there was a cable in the motel room. It looked like it was a TV cable and we had a little portable TV so I wanted to hook it up for the kids. I connected it and over the TV came a radio transmission from the sheriff's office, which I didn't know was right next door. I didn't know where *anything* was at that point so I went to the manager and said, I think there's an emergency call and they're getting the ambulance. He told me to go next door and find out what's going on, so I did. The sheriff deputy promptly threw me into his vehicle and we raced 80 mph down the road about 15 miles.
>
> When we arrived at the scene, the tow truck had a cable going down the side of the mountain. In those days there weren't any guard rails and a car had gone off and was on its roof with a victim inside. The car was unstable and the next ledge went all the way down, about a thousand feet, into the gorge. While they were trying to stabilize the car, I went down that cable, about 100 to 150 feet, with a couple of the fire department guys, hanging onto this cable. I didn't even know if they had supplies but they had IV supplies and some other equipment. When I reached the victim he was unconscious but breathing and vital signs were okay. After stabilizing the car, a Stokes litter was sent down and we got that victim out of there, on a backboard, and put him on that Stokes. We then had to get another cable to take us up the side of the mountain because there was no way to do that without some help. I started an IV on the patient while I was down there and brought him up to the ambulance, there was no helicopter in those days. I went to the nearest hospital with him (55 miles away) where he ultimately died.

The next day was Sunday and I was walking up to church with the kids. On the way, I saw all these people sitting on the bench and they're kind of pointing and talking about me, about the fact that this guy went up and over the bank, which was not something the visiting physicians had ever done. What happened after that was people were able to see that I had some credibility, clinically, because they did not know what an NP was. Before this happened a lot of them wouldn't have come to see an NP, they would go somewhere else to see a physician. So that was a big event that really established my credibility as a provider in the community, and by happenstance it was my first day.

In addition to this description of a trauma situation, Bob narrates a story involving critical medical care:

I remember I had a patient with an MI [myocardial infarction] that I couldn't move anywhere due to a snow storm, so I sat up all night in the clinic ER [emergency room] taking care of that patient and trying to keep her alive and finally got her out.

In another segment of his story Bob describes an urgent obstetrical situation:

We delivered a double-footling breech here with the help of a doctor 55 miles away. He was on the phone and the cord could barely reach to the room and he was telling me what to do and that turned out okay, but it's a pretty scary, not ideal, situation to be in.

Regarding the concept of expert generalist and a rural skillset, Bob had this to say:

We were doing casts, we were doing x-rays, we were doing orthopedics of all kind, minor surgery, a broad scope of skills that are still required, OB [obstetrics] included. We took care of cardiac issues, a lot of mental health issues.

Long and Weinert (1989) identified the concept of having friends and neighbors as patients. This was illustrated in another story Bob narrated:

You get to know these people on a very intimate level. Some of them have relationship problems, some of them have severe medical problems, some of them die. So it never really bothered me to have friends, close friends, who are patients but I think it does limit your social interaction with them because sometimes people don't want those boundaries crossed, and so they're perfectly fine that you know their intimate secrets but they don't want to be at a reception with you and know that you did their pelvic exam, you see, that sort of thing. If they were alcoholic, or if they were somehow impaired or whatever, those elements kept you somewhat aloof from the social aspect of it.

One aim of this book was to bring to light the particular ethics of frontier NP practice. Bob makes several statements that illustrate this concept and tie it to the ethic of stewardship:

I think you're always trying to build in support systems to make sure that you're dealing with the appropriate standard of care for the patients.

Also when discussing the loss of 24/7 medical coverage for the community:

I do understand that it needs to change and the question is, how can it change and not lose that 24/7 care to a population that otherwise would have no access to advanced cardiac life support systems or would have limited access to urgent care. The kind of problems that could be dealt with in a clinic setting and now their needs will either not be met or they'll be met at an ER at four times the cost and *people will die.*

During the interview Bob states that nowadays there are a lot more nonclinical administrators in charge of frontier clinics and that "this makes a difference in terms of how it gets done." In light of the professional challenges he faced as both clinic administrator and health care provider, Bob was asked if he felt it would be done better or worse:

I think it's worse that they're not a clinician because a clinician at least knows that the primary purpose of the institution is to provide care, *to the patient.* And sometimes administration systems exist to support the systems of administration and revenue.

Another concept identified in the literature review is the social capital that frontier NPs bring to their communities. Bob gives some examples of this:

> During a lot of my early days I was intervening in that trauma area because we didn't have any other system to support that . . . we did a lot of training on extrication, we helped get the tools we needed to help get these patients out of those vehicles. We trained a lot of the EMTs.

Social capital is also measured by the number of employed people in a community. As a result of Bob's efforts to improve health care services in the community (mental health, dental, physical therapy) and the infrastructure of the clinic, it became a major employer in the community. At its height, in the early 2000s, the clinic employed 17 people. Since merging with a larger clinic, the number of employees has decreased to less than one third that amount. This is due in part to the decrease in clinic hours and transfer of support staff, such as medical billers and administrative support, to the larger facility.

■ THEMES

Several overall themes emerged from Bob's stories: (a) *charting your own course,* (b) *flying solo,* and (c) *flying by the seat of your pants.* The theme of Bob's personal journey is charting your own course. This theme comprises two subthemes, *taking the road less traveled* and *carving out your own niche,* which are taken directly from the interview text. Bob referenced Robert Frost and stated, "I took the road less traveled, and I did, and I'm all the better for it." When discussing the decision to continue working in an institutional setting or venture into the frontier, Bob stated, "It's hard to carve out your own niche in that environment."

The second theme, flying solo, also comprises two subthemes, *many hats* and *isolation.* The term flying solo is often used to describe a situation in which you are on your own and you have multiple tasks that need to be done, such as flying a plane and navigating at the same time.

The first subtheme, many hats, connoting multiple roles, is similar to Rosenthal's study theme, *fluid role* (1996). However, there are contextual differences between the meaning of many hats in Rosenthal's study and this study. In Rosenthal's study, she referred to rural acute care nurses who worked in several departments during a single shift or to the wide range of tasks they completed during their shift. In this book participants used the term to describe the many roles they filled within their local health care delivery model. This concept is supported by the following exemplars:

- I did all the administration, and that was a challenge in terms of being in a frontier role because you had to administer the clinic, staff it, and provide the care.

- I was also the school nurse . . . the health department really wasn't as integrated then, so we had to deal with immunizations and screenings.

- We taught EMT classes . . . I did house calls . . . covered the jail . . . covered the ambulance . . .

The second subtheme, isolation, is supported by this statement:

You realize working in a frontier area is like being a night nurse and in the middle of the night, when you have something go bad, you have to think, can I deal with this or do I have to call somebody . . . only the difference here is that you couldn't even call anybody . . . it ain't happening here. So you had to deal with it alone and make a decision about what to do.

The third theme, flying by the seat of your pants, connotes entering into a situation that you know little about, but you enter into it anyway, doing the best you can with what you have. It is supported by the following exemplars:

- I really didn't know what was going on. . . . I tried to sort it out and let people know what the issues were.

- I had no idea at that time what would be the preponderance of the care that I would have to give, would it be trauma, medicine, peds, I really didn't know.

- I worked that out in the early days because it wasn't clear how to do it, so we created our own system basically.

- So a lot of that early time, as a provider here, was trying to adapt to these kinds of different needs and developing the skillset you need to do it with . . . because even in the program they really didn't address those kinds of issues, certainly not EMS [emergency medical services] issues.

CONCLUSION

Bob's narrative provides an oral history of the development of a frontier NP practice in one specific state. His story allows NPs to *see* the professional development of NPs over time and within the frontier context. The thick descriptions of his practice experiences allow NPs to reflect on similar experiences they may have had. Bob's narrative also provides an administrative viewpoint and illustrates the power of *policy* as it relates to access to health care in frontier communities.

REFERENCES

Long, K, & Weinert, C. (1989). Rural nursing: developing the theory base. *Scholarly Inquiry for Nursing Practice: An International Journal, 3,* 113-127.

Rosenthal, K. (1996). *Rural nursing: An exploratory narrative description* (Doctoral dissertation). Available from ProQuest Dissertation database (UMI No. 304379526).

5

Ann: A Grow-Your-Own Story

■ OVERVIEW

Ann wears the hats of clinic administrator and health care provider. She is an example of the *grow-your-own* concept:

> I grew up out here, in the northwest, and my father was ill so I decided I wanted to become a nurse and had no idea that was going to be a challenge at all. I became a BSN [bachelor of nursing science] and I had grand ideas that I was going to become an ICU [intensive care unit] nurse and travel the world. I came home for Thanksgiving and met a man who I later married . . . so guess where I started my first practice?

There were no physician offices, clinics, or hospitals to work at; therefore, Ann had to find creative ways to use her new nursing skills:

> I became an EMT [emergency medical technician], I taught childbirth classes, and did anything I thought was related to nursing. I did it, promoted it and used those hours to renew my RN license.

It was the late 1970s and people were beginning to hear about the nurse practitioner (NP) role. Ann and a group of community members tried to recruit an NP to their community, but found a PA (physician assistant) to take the job instead:

> He practiced for 2 years to meet the requirements of the National Health Service Corp loan repayment program, then he left. We then tried to merge with other agencies (100–150 miles in any direction) and one of them sent a visiting doctor. . . . We'd have someone here for a while, then the politics would change and he or she would leave.

As a result of unreliable and interrupted access to health care in her community, Ann went back to school and got her NP certification. She started a community clinic on a shoestring budget, and had little or no money for equipment:

> We didn't have personal protective equipment that looked like what they had in the hospital, but we had farm safety goggles, and we had raingear.

Ann had been one of the few nurses in her community. There had never been an established medical office; therefore, no one in the community had ever been trained to work in one:

> You have no staff to recruit, if there are RNs out here, they're out here for some purpose other than health care or they want a wage, which is something *to this day* that I can't offer. So we hire bar maids and grocery clerks and train them to our needs.

Additionally, there were no funds to hire ancillary staff even if there were qualified people available:

> . . . so you have to wear many hats. You're the housekeeper, carpenter, the plumber, the repairman, because there's nobody to call in. We're getting more and more people and now I actually have people I can call to work on the plumbing, it's a wonderfully federal-funded thing, but I still do a lot of things here.

Eventually, the community became a taxing district which provided tax revenue to help fund access to stable health care. Through community efforts and grant funds, a medical clinic came into being.

■ CONCEPTS

A review of literature indicates that one of the main differences between rural nursing and frontier nursing is the number and acuity level of emergency patients that are seen. When asked to relate a story that paints a picture of what it's like to be a frontier NP, Ann thought this over for a while and then responded with a story involving emergency care:

> This guy came in, he had been out . . . and he came in with part of his face peeled off, literally peeled from mid-eye to ear. He came to the clinic and refused to go on, didn't have

money, didn't have transportation, didn't have a good car, maybe didn't have a license, I didn't know. So I made him sign his life away (consent to treatment, and refusal to seek a higher level of care), and I said, okay, I'll try to put you back together but you have to know, this is beyond anything that I think I'm capable of doing. So 6 hours, several bathroom breaks, Vicodin for him and Advil for me (due to bending over for so long), I had him back together. He looks pretty good, he has function, he talks, and he's satisfied.

When asked if her NP program provided education on emergency care skills, Ann relays a story that also includes the concept of the art of frontier NP practice:

No. No, it's all learned on the job. And trauma is so different for each person. For example, the other day we had a child that had been cut by . . . it was a deep cut, it had probably nicked an artery, and there was lots of blood involved. We probably could have sewn him up but he was so shocky, so traumatized, and the adults were so traumatized by the whole affair that it was not in our best interest or the client's best interest to sew him up. So, when do you sew up a face and when do you refer a little cut? It's an art.

Working with trauma victims often involves working with local emergency medical services (EMS) systems. When asked about managing trauma victims, Ann explained some of the inner workings of the EMS system in her community:

I depend on the EMS, I wouldn't live here, and I couldn't survive, if I didn't have EMS because I *cannot* sustain a life here. My IV bags out-date, I'm lucky to have two IV bags and once I'm done with those two then there's hell to pay, so if I really need lots of volume I'm not going to last very long. I can't carry ACLS [advanced cardiac life support] drugs because they're too expensive, they out-date too fast. So I rely on EMS for drugs.

When asked about the availability of an all-volunteer EMS system, Ann provides this example:

It's all volunteer and so much of the time there is no response. It's summer they're gone, they're vacationing, they're harvesting, they're just not available, so we go the next community, 30 miles away and they're also harvesting and farming. That community has two EMT 2s (their scope is higher than EMTs), one worked for the government, but the government office closed so we don't even have that resource. So then we can call on the next community down (70 miles away) or we can call in an air ambulance if they're available, which has a 20- to 30-minute estimated time of arrival, but you need fire department and other personnel to land them. Last weekend, someone, who has renal failure and congestive heart failure, he's very ill, he called 911 because he was vomiting after his last chemo therapy and "he's going downhill rapidly" according to the call. It happened to be on my day off but somehow I got involved anyway. There were no EMTs to respond so after about an hour a couple of first-responders got to the scene, assessed the patient, decided he didn't need an air ambulance and he came to the clinic.

In Bob's state, the clinic had to have an alternative-base-station designation to allow EMS personnel to transport patients to Bob's clinic. I asked Ann if the EMS regional oversight committee took issue with the transport of some emergency patients to her clinic:

They are the one who tells them to bring the patients here. If you take that client who had the nausea from his chemotherapy, to the hospital (approximately 100 miles away), you take my EMTs out of the community for 6 hours, that's a staff of two in the back, one in the front, probably a few first-responders, so that's four EMS personnel, and that's the ambulance. I have six responders and that leaves me one and one backup ambulance for six hours because the round trip takes 4 to 5 hours plus another 2 hours to transfer the client, paperwork, clean the rig and get it ready for the next run. Six hours is the minimum that an ambulance run can happen. You leave my community open for a gun-shot wound with no response.

Frontier communities lack access to mental health services. Ann talked about the impact this lack of services has on her frontier community:

I have a bipolar patient, who is identified by the insurance company as one of their top spenders, but I can't justify the cost of tele-medicine to show people how psychotic the patient is, so I just have to handle the psychotic episodes, and they're very expensive to the community, not just the health care system. Everybody gets involved, the sheriff, the people in the community, *everybody* was in my office saying you gotta do something about this, but what am *I* going to do? . . . I finally get her sent for an evaluation but it happens there's no pharmacy open at the moment, so they send her back with three days' worth of medicine. Well she gets back and she doesn't have meds and I don't have the meds, so I have to order the meds, so yeah. That's when I really wanted, *needed*, tele-medicine, I can't tell you how come I can't have it, it hasn't worked, and I did my entire thesis on it.

Dr. Mary Wakefield, deputy secretary of the U.S. Department of Health and Human Services (Wakefield, 2014), has stated that tele-health was the future of health care in rural areas of the country. In light of this stance, Ann was questioned further:

I wrote a grant to get broadband; the only reason I can justify keeping it, is that I have EMRs [electronic medical records], it's in the *cloud* and so I can justify keeping it for an outrageous amount of money, for my community. But I can't hook up with anybody. Who practices tele-health in this state, no one. I can hook up with next state over, but who's going pay for it? And you gotta have somebody *to* call in, they are basically on-call waiting for us to have a case, well I can't afford to have anyone on-call for my tele-health. I wanted to do tele-health with just mental health, they don't have a psychiatric mental health nurse practitioner. I did find someone, but they could only Skype in and that's illegal, that's not even HIPAA [Health Insurance Portability and Accountability Act] compliant, but it's tele-health. But I can't get it to happen in *my* clinic. We were part of a year-long study with one of the universities, because that made sense, they do tele-health. And it's another one of those . . . I can't tell you all of details of why it was that it couldn't work here. We didn't have the $50,000 for the transmission equipment, so we could write a grant for the equipment but then we need multi-specialty care, we don't need just one kind of care, but I don't have the patient numbers to make it worthwhile for them.

Ann goes on to discuss personal challenges related to frontier NP practice. Two concepts identified by Long and Weinert (1989) were evident in Ann's narrative. The first involved having family and friends as patients:

That's why I wear scrubs, it's putting on my different hat. Everybody's your family and friend. You know intimate details about people that you shouldn't know. . . . They see you in the grocery store and start right in with their medical problems and I have to remind them that I'm not wearing my scrubs and, would you take that (whatever the problem or issue was) to the clinic. It's always your family and friends, so . . . you care for them and then you deal with the rest of the junk.

Long and Weinert (1989) also identified characteristics of rural dwellers. They found that rural dwellers tend to identify the ability to work with being healthy. They also tend to put off seeking care until their work is done. This segment of Ann's narrative exemplifies this concept:

This guy came in with a tib/fib fracture and he'd been on a horse. The horse ran his foot into the fence and it just twisted it backward but the stirrup brought it back into alignment. So I said, why didn't you come in earlier and he said, well, they were still working . . . and there was nobody to drive me and if I got off the horse it would have hurt. So he just stayed on the horse until they were through . . . and 5 hours later he came into the clinic and wanted me to fix his fracture. You know, that's frontier life.

The concept of seasonal population variations has been identified as a personal challenge to NPs practicing in some frontier settings:

Rural used to be all about industry, we're not about industry anymore; we're about tourism. So we have, on major holiday weekends, an influx of about three to five thousand people.

Ann spoke about the rural skillset and competencies required to work in this type of setting:

Nursing school doesn't teach you how to run a business. We don't have a hierarchy, we have a lateral system because none of us work full time, we're all here part time, so

everybody needs to know how to turn the water off when it
floods, everybody needs to know the management system,
everybody. I have a limited x-ray permit, but we're afraid the
regulations are going to change and we won't even have
that. How do you get lab techs? You can't ask somebody else
to do it. If it needs to be done you'd better learn how to do it
because there's nobody else.

The concept of solo practice was also evident in the literature review
and Ann discusses why it is usually the case:

We had a second provider, through the NHSC [National
Health Service Corps] loan repayment program, but when
that ended he left. The population numbers haven't changed
so paying two provider salaries was too difficult. So then we
had to recruit *again*, which always takes about a year at the
bare minimum because people just don't have the skillset, or
they come here and they're frightened immediately because
you tell them what they're going to be doing.

Currently, in order to achieve 2-hour staffing, Ann and her relief
provider each work in the clinic during office hours and on call after office hours; they do this for 5 to 14 days straight. Due to the challenges in
just finding a relief provider, she worries what will happen to the clinic
as she nears retirement age.

The concept of social capital was discussed in the literature review.
Ann was asked about the social capital she may bring to her community:

There's only so many people who are doers and if you're a
doer you do everything to point that you burn out. I used
to be involved everywhere, but I'm currently withdrawn
from everything as a self-protection mode. . . . I think we
bring a lot of social capital because we bring our educational
background to the entire community.

As we heard from Bob, federal policy has a profound effect on frontier health care. Ann is also the clinic administrator and has this to say:

Government policies are another thing, they write all these
policies. I am such an idealist, I got started on this whole
trip [NP career] because the government said that NPs were
going to fill in in rural areas. Well, I happen to be vested
in a very rural area, but then there wasn't funding for it.

Then they say you know, put in a rural health clinic, but now they're not funding it, but we have more and more requirements like EMRs and electronic billing that require software agreements, licenses and network maintenance, which aren't necessarily covered in start-up grants.

Despite her frustration regarding governmental policy shifts, the last concept comes from Ann herself, when she discusses the political nature of her frontier role and the importance of networking with political allies:

You have to get politicians involved. I have politicians tour my clinic yearly, I personally know them, I go talk to them, I've been to DC; I've stood on the Capitol steps because that's what you need to do to get your voice heard. If you don't make your voice heard nothing ever happens, and that's why I have a clinic that's beautiful now, because they said yes to the grant, they were willing to co-fund it, they knew us personally. People don't understand those personal connections, like attending rural health clinic meetings and knowing who is in your political set, that is extremely important, that's how we got our taxing district, that's how we got our supervising physician, and how we got laws changed, *extremely* important.

■ THEMES

Four overall themes emerged from Ann's narrative: (a) *it doesn't work here*, (b) *out on a limb*, (c) *there's an art to it*, and (d) *reciprocity of care*. Embedded in the first theme is the idea that outsiders, or people who live in larger population centers, think that it *does* work here. This is akin to taking for granted that systems developed for use in nonfrontier settings will work in frontier communities. In addition to the inability to access tele-health, other communication systems may be inaccessible at times:

Cell phones, yes everyone has them but they don't always work, there are pockets where they don't work. If the power goes down, your communications go down, people can't communicate when it's down. The fire department has radios, but it's all communicated through one town, over 70 miles away, through one 911 system that we have. There's no local control so if anything affects those towers, like an earthquake, we're in deep trouble.

While telling another story, she interjects:

Just the distance makes things so difficult, things that people just don't think of.

And when discussing why normal procedures and protocols don't work in her setting:

I get tired of explaining to people why it just doesn't work here.

The second theme, out on a limb, refers to how NPs may need to manage situations they are not necessarily prepared for:

Someone came in with a head wound that looked great when I opened it up; it was only 6 to 8 inches long. And then I started washing it. He had, what turned out to be, three severed arteries, so I could not clear the field to tie one off. As soon as I started to say oh no, in my own mind, *I* felt like I was going to pass out so it was *me* walking around with ice packs in my arm pits and sticking my head under the faucet, telling his friend, *hold pressure, hold pressure*, oh no, what am I going to do! So I just sutured the wound together, whipped it together, to try to get a tamponade, put an ice pack and a diaper on his wound to vasoconstrict it, I put all the Epi I had in it, that didn't completely vasoconstrict it but I got enough ice on it that he quit *squirting*, he started *oozing*, so I put a diaper and a few more ice packs on his wound. Because it was the middle of the night and there were no EMTs, he decided to drive to the ER [emergency room] and he survived and he did just fine.

The third theme, there's an art to it, refers not only explicitly to the phrase Ann used when discussing whether you stitch up a face or sew a finger, but implicitly when she talks about redirecting patients who would discuss their medical problems in public. Embedded in this theme is the notion that there is an *art* to maintaining not only patient confidentiality in small communities, but your own as well.

The fourth theme, reciprocity of care, refers to the reciprocal nature of caring in a frontier community. It is embedded in the concept of having friends and neighbors as patients. While you care for or treat them, they also care about you. This is exemplified in one of Ann's stories:

> One day I had a bladder infection and my gossiping relative found out that I had home visits to do that day. So everywhere I went they all said, "Would you like to use the bathroom?" the first thing when I got there, because my relative had told them about my problem. So, it's interesting, you're isolated but you're not.

■ CONCLUSION

Ann used the phrase "many hats" in her narrative. This is one of the subthemes in Bob's story. Ann uses this phrase to connote and delineate the different roles she has in the community. This is exemplified when she discusses wearing scrubs to delineate her role as NP to her patients.

Ann's commitment to both her patients and her community is evident. Through Ann's narrative the reader can also see the strong commitment she has to the nursing profession. She demonstrates nursing leadership and has taken her voice to Capitol Hill for the benefit of her community and her profession.

REFERENCES

Long, K, & Weinert, C. (1989). Rural nursing: Developing the theory base. *Scholarly Inquiry for Nursing Practice: An International Journal, 3,* 113–127.

Wakefield, M. (2014, July). *The Affordable Care Act: Implications for rural health and rural nursing.* Keynote speech presented at the International Rural Health and Rural Nursing Research Conference, Bozeman, MT.

6

Jim: A Midlife Transition

■ OVERVIEW

In his late forties, Jim enrolled in a family nurse practitioner (FNP) program. He was chief flight nurse at a prestigious medical center and enjoyed the work, but felt he needed to widen his career choices, "even though I'm in relatively good health you're only going to be able to get in and out of a helicopter for a certain amount of time." The FNP program had a rural focus, but Jim had not given any thought to rural or frontier practice:

> I never really thought about that, I knew at some point I
> would probably transition into an NP practice, whether
> that would be emergency medicine, urgent care, or family
> practice. I never really had a thought that this is what I was
> going to do when I started the program.

After graduation, Jim worked part time at an urgent care clinic. During a trip to . . . on a ski vacation, Jim and his wife started thinking that they might like to buy a vacation home in . . . because they really liked the area. On the way home, they discussed it further:

> We are both in our fifties so we kind of started thinking
> about making the move sooner rather than later. So I went
> home and kind of just did an online search, just out of
> curiosity, and *this* particular job was posted 2 hours prior
> to me looking. I was working here less than 2 months later.
> But I never had a vision of, okay, I'm going to go out and
> practice in a rural setting, in the middle of nowhere, and be
> the provider that people looked to.

This job is a family practice clinic attached to a 10-bed critical access hospital (CAH), which includes two emergency department beds. Jim works with two physicians and two physician assistants. Until recently, he had been the only NP, but now there is a pediatric NP in the clinic 1 day per week. This now makes a total of six providers (a mix of full and part time) to care for 2,500 residents in this vast community. Jim is unaware of any specific grant funding that supports the hospital:

> The hospital is a not-for-profit, I don't believe they have grant funding, but we have a very high Medicare population, and this is something I learned about here, with CAHs, Medicare is actually a better payer source than private insurance.

Jim has practiced in the frontier setting for more than 2 years now. When asked if he was surprised by any facet of his new role, he had this to say:

> I didn't really think about how closely or how intimate you get into somebody's life with their health care. It's more than just seeing patients every day, it's that we see people continually, we get to know them a little bit more. It's a little more personal than it would be if you were working in a larger place.

The challenges of providing 24/7 health care coverage to a community were illustrated by Bob's and Ann's stories. Jim's situation is different; he is not the sole provider for an entire community. Call duties are shared within the group:

> That was one of things I started looking at because in my prior job I was chief flight nurse for 5 years and part of that job was call every fourth week.
>
> I was on call 24/7 for 7 days and got minimal pay, something like $2 per hour.
>
> Even though 99% of the time it was just phone stuff, it still limited what you could do. I didn't want to ever be on call again but the system here makes it much more palatable. I take call one night per week and one weekend per month.

There can be a fairly high turnover rate of providers in frontier settings, but both Jim and his wife have integrated into the community and seem happy with their decision to move here. I asked Jim if he was planning to stay:

> The transition to frontier life has been easy, I mean quite easy. At this point, I don't see us doing anything different. As long as things stay the way they are now, *here*, you

know the working relationship that we all have, and if this hospital stays solvent, yeah. There's always things that can change, but yeah.

■ CONCEPTS

When asked what it's like to be a frontier NP, Jim narrates a story that illustrates both the need for mental health services in frontier settings and the intimate nature of frontier NP practice:

There is an adolescent in our community who had recently undergone a lot of family trauma and grief. About 3 months later I started seeing him for depression. So, I went through the whole process, started him on anti-depressants, started having him in frequently, had him see a psychiatrist through tele-health, who kind of helped me manage the medications for the patient. I saw him again 4 to 5 months ago in the clinic and could tell he was really depressed. I said, if you ever decide to hurt yourself or do anything, you need to call me. I gave him my cell phone number along with my home number. I also gave him the number of the crisis counselor and suicide prevention hotline. I said, I don't do this often for people but I want you to call me. I was on call one weekend, I was driving from my house to the clinic, and I get this phone call and it's an 800 number I've never seen. This lady gets on the phone and said, are you . . . and I said yes, and she said I'm . . . from the suicide hotline and I've got . . . on the line. I was like, wow, okay. So she puts . . . on the phone and I convinced him to come into the hospital. The patient was at home, alone in a room, contemplating suicide. I said, please tell me you'll come in to see me and he said, yes I will and he came in. The patient had made a plan to take every pill in the house. He had made a *definitive* plan, not only had he thought about it, but decided, this is what I am going to do. So, I got him admitted to a pediatric mental health facility. The patient completed both an in-patient and out-patient program. I sent him a card saying hang in there, and he replied with a letter essentially telling me that if it weren't for me he wouldn't be alive. You know that's kind of the unique position that you're in, working in a frontier community, it's not real often that you get to be that directly involved with, especially someone that age, who probably would have taken all those pills and killed himself.

This brought up another ethical concept regarding the on-call responsibilities of a frontier NP: in Jim's case, the ethics of availability.

You know, it's one of those things, the self-responsibility. I don't want to be somewhere without cell service for an hour and someone's here in critical condition, *that's just wrong.* It's wrong for the patient, it's wrong for the community.

Having friends and neighbors as patients is another recurring concept in the literature. Jim has not lived in his community as long as Bob and Ann have; however, he still has experience with this aspect of frontier NP practice:

I lived in one particular town for 16 years and worked in the EMS [emergency medical services] system there for 6 years, so I knew a lot of people and had to take care of friends and family. So it's one of those things that you kind of keep in the back of your mind but till you're faced with it, it's not that big of a deal, you just don't think about it. It's not something I dwell on, it's one of those things coming from my background and what I've done, it doesn't matter who it is, you just get in there and do the best you can and take care of it.

The fire station and ambulance bay are in close proximity to the clinic. Local EMS are provided through volunteers, and the ambulance offers only basic life support (BLS) services. Jim was asked if the EMS were integrated with the clinic or the CAH:

Technically there's really no integration, but we have a working relationship. We have no oversight of them; they have a separate medical director who is not from the community. The board of medicine has regulations that do not technically allow me to give orders over the radio and I cannot be a medical director for the EMS program because I am not a physician or a PA [physician assistant]. Now there's really not a lot I could order them to do anyway because they're a BLS system and they really can't do a whole lot to begin with. They can't start IVs in the field so when the patient comes in here, to the emergency department it's like you're getting them from a first responder situation. . . . As far as I know, there is no formal way to integrate RNs or NPs into the EMS system in this state. The ambulance delivers the patients to the emergency department and we take over from there.

Jim has brought the skills derived from his previous trauma experience to his new position:

I am now the trauma director for the hospital. I have also taught classes for the EMS folks. Since I've been here, I've intubated six people in the emergency department. Prior to me coming here, the director of nursing told me nobody had been intubated by a provider in this hospital in over 10 years. Before I came here they had no ventilator. I convinced them to purchase not only a ventilator that we can use temporarily in the hospital, but one that we can use for transport as well. So for all intents and purposes, I can confidently say that I have at least elevated the level of critical care that people get in this community.

Jim has added to the social capital in his new community in other ways as well:

By way of my position as trauma director, I am involved in a community outreach program. Next spring I am planning to do a ghost op. Right before prom or graduation you do a mock crash and then you bring in a helicopter and you do the whole thing to let people know, this is what it's like when you get in a bad car accident. The other thing I've done is written several articles in the paper on health topics like sinusitis and things like that. I've also been approached about joining a mental health committee, for lack of a better phrase. They're going to look at the mental health capabilities of the valley and see if there are ways to improve it. . . . I'm not a mental health professional, it's probably one of my weakest areas.

■ THEMES

The theme of Jim's personal journey is *transition*. He uses this term several times throughout his narrative. Jim transitioned into a new career as an FNP, a new job, and into a new community and a new lifestyle, one that is in the frontier.

The second theme in Jim's story, *a different mindset*, is taken directly from the interview text. This theme indicates that Jim has come to discover that there *is* a difference between frontier NP practice and practice in a more urban area. Jim is asked to relate what it is like to be a frontier NP:

> I come from a background of critical care. I quite honestly have probably seen the worst that you can see happen to the human body. *A lot*, I mean I've seen a lot of it. Out here you kind of have to have a different mindset dealing with one, the population, and two, your lack of resources.

Near the end of the interview, Jim was asked if he wanted to add anything else as far as frontier NP practice was concerned:

> Yes, I think one of the things that is really key in frontier practice for *any* provider, regardless whether it's a physician, NP, PA, it doesn't really matter, anybody who's overseeing somebody's care, you really have to have a different mindset on how you do things in a setting like this. For example, someone may come in with knee pain and you can look at that knee, you can assess the knee and say, okay, maybe they're going to need an MRI. In most places you automatically refer him or her to an orthopedist, that person is going to go right to an orthopedist; you're not going to do anything else. Out here you have to have a different mindset because, number one, everything's not close, and two, you can't readily have specialty physicians to take care of patients. So you really have to concentrate more on a good physical exam, a good history, and then think; okay, is this test that I'm thinking about doing appropriate, is it cost effective, and how is it going to affect the person?

■ CONCLUSION

Jim's story is quite different from Bob's and Ann's. Jim's extensive trauma experiences, in addition to support staff and more sophisticated equipment, give him the confidence to handle emergent situations. When asked what being a frontier NP is like, Ann and Bob both responded with stories of emergency situations. Jim answered with a story of human struggle and the intimate bond between frontier practitioner and patient.

Jim's story also gives us a different perspective of frontier NP practice. Rather than a solo practitioner working in geographic and professional isolation, Jim's experience of practicing in a medical clinic attached to a CAH would appear to be an effective health care delivery model in his particular setting. This model may also ameliorate some of the personal challenges of working in the frontier, such as (a) professional isolation, (b) scare resources, and (c) heavy on-call commitments.

Jim's community is fortunate to have a person with his experience and professionalism. Both Jim and his wife have added to the social capital in their community and have been rewarded with a sense of belonging and being *home*.

7

Pam: The Traveler

◾ OVERVIEW

Pam lives in a community that is 80% Native American. There is a reservation 14 miles from her community with a small hospital and ambulance service. However, if you are not Native American, it is difficult to avail yourself of their services. Pam came to the frontier by way of marriage. She grew up in a metropolitan area but always wanted to live in a rural setting:

> I love looking at the wildlife, I love watching the seasons change, I love waving to the farmers when they're planting or harvesting their crops, I don't know, I just love it. I also love rural health. People in rural America will help you. I have lived in other places and it's not the same as when you live in rural areas, it's just, people trust each other. . . .

For the past year, Pam has worked as a nurse practitioner (NP) in a physician-owned clinic in her frontier community. Prior to this, Pam had traveled out of her community to work in other frontier settings. Travel meant being on call, which usually entailed being away from home for several days at a time:

> You can't sleep because you're not in your own bed. So you're lying there and you think, I've got to get to sleep! Finally, you fall asleep around 2:30 in the morning and at 3 o'clock somebody calls, it's the ER [emergency room], you've got 20 minutes to get there, maximum. So you try to look like a person when you roll out of your motel room. Of course, it's totally cold out so your car's half frozen. I tell you, I finally got a car starter. Before that I would have to go out there and crank it over and hope it would start. So then

you'd make it to the hospital or the clinic, you'd get out of your car, and you're frozen [chuckle].

Pam's sense of humor is evident as she continues:

And then, you get there and this little boy had an *earache*. You examine the child and tell the parent what to do and you smile [laughter] and that's all that you can do, then you start the whole cycle over again. Okay, now the car's kind of warmed up, you go back to the hotel room, after you dictate, of course. You go back to the hotel and you can't sleep and when you do get sleep, it's time to go to work, and you realize you forgot to eat the day before so you're really hungry!

For a while Pam had worked in a frontier community approximately 110 miles west of her home. She worked for a clinic that was attached to a critical access hospital (CAH) and a skilled nursing facility. This required an extended daily commute (along with some weekend call), which could be dangerous in harsh weather: "You have to be prepared, but I loved it, absolutely loved it."

■ CONCEPTS

The concept of limited resources and support in frontier settings is evident in the literature. The CAH was a satellite facility of a larger health care organization. One aspect of working within that system was the amount of support Pam had. For example, if Pam were called to the ER for a medical emergency, she had physician backup by telephone: "They'd talk you right through it. They were just there for you, all the time."

Even with telephone support, there are issues when dealing with trauma patients, particularly managing multiple trauma patients when you're alone:

It's a nightmare. The patient's family doesn't understand why the other patient might be more important than their family member, or whatever. And it's hard to have enough supplies on hand because they cost so much. People don't understand things like that.

Pam received support in other areas as well:

I'm not comfortable with x-rays and so, they sent me down to . . . and I spent some time with the radiologist. Out here the x-ray can be a very valuable tool but they have actually cut x-ray services in most of the clinics where I used to work. The hospitals make more money if you have to send the patients all the way over there.

The lack of mental health services in frontier communities is evident both in the literature and in the previous stories. This concept is woven throughout Pam's narrative:

I see a lot of depression, a lot of anxiety. It's just, there is no mental health provider here. I wish I had gotten a psych NP license because it's so overwhelming. I've taken a lot of CEU [continuing education unit] courses and I read a lot about it. We have an addiction/recovery worker here and he's been helpful as well.

Pam alludes to the stigma that mental health patients may face in frontier communities:

When I worked in . . . I talked them into getting a counselor in there, it worked so well. His office was next to mine so when you went down the hall you couldn't tell if the person was going to my office or his office, which was excellent, it worked so well. But then the grant manager switched administrators and she didn't think it was necessary to provide the service. *Why is a human mind not part of the body;* where do people get that, I don't understand it.

Pam then relates a story that exemplifies the need for mental health services in the frontier:

I was called to the ER for a 9-year-old girl who had been raped. It was a tragedy, just horrible. She was sitting there with her little bunny socks on and I thought, dear God, how am I going to help this girl. It was just; that was the worst case I've even seen. It's a shame, just a shame. The poor little girl didn't know what was going on so I sent her to the psychiatric unit for observation. I thought, she's going to need help and I thought, where are your parents? You know, they're young people, it's just so sad. They need mental health; mental health would be a good thing.

This brought up the concepts of confidentiality in a frontier community and having family and friends as patients:

Privacy rights (HIPAA [Health Insurance Portability and Accountability Act]), are not realistic at all [laughs]. All people have to do is look at whose house you're parked in front of, or, was that so-and-so's car at the clinic, then the rumors start. I've had people pull their shirts up to show me this bump they've got and I'm like, in the drugstore. It's like *really*, why don't you come and see me later, okay [laughs]. As far as having family and friends as patients, most of the time it's very rewarding.

The theme *reciprocity of care* emerged from Ann's story when she discussed her home care patients offering the use of their bathrooms. This concept is evident is Pam's narrative as well. She was on call, in a motel room, over the Thanksgiving holiday. She relates what she found when she returned to her room after an ER call out:

There was food on every open space, on the nightstand, everywhere in the motel room. Somebody brought me buffalo steak [laughs], you know, to me, that was just the nicest thing.

She goes on to say:

I would get stuck and they would come right over and pull me out. . . . You tend to make friends, so you always have a place to stay if something goes wrong. I have a patient who used to bring me cardboard to put in front of my radiator so my motor wouldn't freeze. It's just a nice feeling that even though I don't live here but I work here, the people would be so nice to me, you know, it fills your heart with good and it makes you want to pass it around.

The frontier skillset was another concept discussed in the literature review. An additional skill may be the ability to look beyond the obvious for answers to patient problems, particularly when resources are limited and the population is vulnerable:

I had a guy come in who stank! I thought I was going to die. It was his foot, it stank and it hurt. He had a cast on his left foot and it had been on for a long time. What happened, why are you wearing a cast? "Oh, I fell I think, and they put it on, it's been a couple of months." I said well, it's got to come off. He said, "Oh my, you can't take it off." I said, I think we can, we'll try the best we can. "No, they took my boot when they put the cast on." So, that was the reason he wouldn't have it removed, he didn't have a boot. So we went to the rummage box and found the man a pair of boots which resolved the situation. But when he came in I just had thought, what is wrong with this man, he stank. He hadn't thought about how they helped his foot, he just thought that they stole his boot!

■ THEMES

Two overall themes emerge from Pam's narrative: *shifting sands* and *a barren health care landscape*. The first theme, shifting sands, refers not only to the fact that Pam has had to shift jobs, but the fact that this occurred partly in response to shifting government priorities. A barren health care landscape refers both to the lack of health care providers/facilities in frontier communities and her drive through barren landscapes to get to her patients.

Shifting federal priorities and funding schemes have been concepts evident in the previous stories. When asked if she would recommend frontier practice, Pam had this to say:

I would say be very careful. There are a limited number of jobs. It's like a politician who gets a term in office, the jobs that are available last for only a short time because the politics change.

Pam explains why she lost one of her frontier NP positions:

They took the funding from my clinic in . . . and gave it to . . . where they felt it would do more good. But they already had a hospital down there, but all the people in . . . had was the clinic, that's it. Those people now have nothing, absolutely nothing. To me that's backwards. The larger cities like . . . they have a community health center that was just built. They already had a hospital and numerous clinics and now they have a health center. They have *nothing* out here, *nothing*. We don't even have 911, I mean we have it, but it has not been certified by the state, so we're all alone.

The term *barren* may be used to indicate that something is lacking. Pam's last statement supports the fact that health care is lacking in the communities she has served. In fact, Pam's motivation to enter an NP program was the lack of health care in her community:

> I just thought it would be good for the community and myself because, like I said, we have *no one* here . . . when you live it, it's different, people die and that's not good. And when the lights go off at the clinic [i.e., if the clinic closes], I'm here, that's it.

When asked if there was anything more she wanted to say, Pam's humor was again evident: "Not right at this time, but thank you for the offer."

■ CONCLUSION

Bob's and Ann's stories allude to the concept of rotating physicians and visiting health care providers in frontier communities; Pam's story provides insight from that perspective, a traveler's perspective. Her story provides a narrative of her experiences spanning a frontier region rather than a single community. Pam states that despite the need for frontier NPs, at this point in time, she regrets her decision to become an NP and cannot look back on a satisfying career. "You know, I could have been director of the nursing home, stayed home and made more money, but this type of work *is* more rewarding."

8

Sue: A Corporate–Frontier Challenge

■ OVERVIEW

Sue grew up in mostly small towns and hails from a family of physicians. After receiving her RN license, she practiced in several locations that included a large metropolitan hospital and a small-town community hospital. She worked primarily intensive care and in the emergency room (ER). One of her moves was to a community in a neighboring state:

> I heard about a program in. . . . They were using RNs on
> their ambulance, as paramedics basically. So we moved
> there and stayed for almost 2 years in which I gained a lot
> of experience in the ER and did a few ambulance runs. The
> nurses were a union organization and would not allow
> the 24-hour shifts with 12-hour regular pay and 12-hour
> standby pay, similar to the ambulance crew schedule. As
> this had not been negotiated before RNs were hired, along
> with a substantial outlay of money, the program never flew,
> because the hospital was not going to pay RNs overtime on
> a 24-hour workday.

While working there, Sue was diagnosed with a chronic medical condition that greatly affected her ability to work. To be closer to family for support, she, her husband, and small children moved to their current community. Sue's medical condition stabilized and she started working at the local clinic 1 day per week to get her "feet in the door." Ten years later, she decided to enroll in a nurse practitioner (NP) program where she received a master's degree.

The community clinic was owned by a group of physicians who staffed the clinic part time. Once Sue had her NP license, she was hired to provide service as an NP and has worked several days per week in that role. A few years ago, the physician group made the decision to sell the clinic to a corporate health care organization, which is located in one of the state's largest cities, 150 miles away.

As noted in the introduction to Part II, narratives are a snapshot in time. The clinic has undergone significant change as a result of the change in ownership. At times, change brings conflict. Depending upon one's perspective, change can also have both favorable and unfavorable consequences. These changes and their impact on her practice are the focus of Sue's narrative.

▪ CONCEPTS

The concept of a frontier culture was discussed in Chapter 1 and examined in Chapter 3. Sue feels that corporate America does not have a basic understanding of the culture of frontier communities:

> My biggest struggle right now is that there doesn't seem
> to be anyone in this whole, huge corporate thought
> process who is willing to look at what it means to a small
> community, when even little changes are made to the
> delivery of health care. For example, we've been told
> that we can't put any local communication on our clinic
> communication board. The corporation does not seem
> to care what the communication board means to a small
> community and that it is an important way we communicate
> with each other. No one took the time to see how this might
> impact our clinic or that it might produce significant ill will.
> No person came and asked us, they just said, this is our
> policy and only what we okay can go on the board. It seems
> like a small thing, but it's one of those types of things that
> undermine trust in a small-town setting. There doesn't seem
> to be an effort to understand the small-town culture and
> that's more frustrating to me than anything.

Prior to the change in clinic ownership, Sue would overlap a day a week with one of the physicians. This enhanced collaborative practice and gave her a sounding board that decreased her sense of professional isolation. Due to physician turnover, Sue now works days where there is no overlap of provider services. As a result of the change in ownership, the clinic now has an electronic medical record (EMR) system that allows for integration with the larger facility in a different location. The clinic is small and only has room for one provider computer and dictation center, and Sue states that it is not feasible for more than one provider to work at the same time. Therefore, to enhance professional collaboration, Sue is now a preceptor for NP students from various programs around the country. So far she has been a preceptor for four students:

> Although I'm a very independent person, I miss the camaraderie of having other people to interact with. You learn so much. Currently my student is an ER nurse and she is a *delight*. It's great to have someone to talk things over with. While you're explaining why you do certain things, you're validating what you're thinking and clarifying your own thought processes.

Although the EMR has decreased the availability of local professional collaboration, it has enhanced distance collaboration:

> I can message a cardiologist, tell them briefly what's going on, I can run an EKG on our old machine and scan it in, have it in media on the computer, and say, can you look at this and tell me what's going on. They'll get back to me, often in the same day. That did not usually happen prior to the EMR. That piece of being able to actually communicate with specialty providers, that I have a collaborative relationship with, is awesome.

Sue gives another example of how integration has enhanced her ability to coordinate care:

> There was a young female patient who wanted to see me but she lives in . . . [over 100 miles away]. She was having a lot of medical problems, migraine headaches, fatigue, and generally not feeling well. She has a history of some liver problems so I decided to order a complete abdominal ultrasound. She had the ultrasound and some lab work done in. . . . I got all those results back an hour later. It was *boom*, right here. I was able to call her and say, everything looks okay, and I'm over 100 miles away. So that is one of the good things.

Integration has not helped in the area of mental health. Sue states that there is no real mental health support system in her community. Many of the patients have Medicaid and many of the mental health pro- viders won't take Medicaid, "so we're kind of stuck out in the middle of no-man's land without it." She hopes that this will change as there is talk of tele-health coming to the community. Although tele-health is something she feels the community could benefit from, she's not sure if people would use it for mental health:

> You're not person to person, you're having an office visit that takes place over video. The personal becomes more impersonal. When you're right there, face to face, you can touch them and just let them know you care, that's a much better practice especially in a frontier community.

Sue said they are not integrated with the local emergency medical services (EMS) system either. The EMS utilize a local ambulance or an air ambulance to transport patients 55 miles to the nearest rural hospital, or 150 miles to the nearest trauma center. Sue keeps current her advanced cardiac life support (ACLS) certification just in case, but states that the clinic does not keep ACLS medications on hand:

> We have an AED [automated external defibrillator], some medications and oxygen. In the past, we have had a full emergency kit of medications, supplies and equipment, but to keep all those medicines is very expensive and have been rarely used in 30 years.

This brought up the issue of being on call. Sue states that since the sale of the clinic she does not have official call time but since she's the only local health care provider, she receives calls at home:

> It's interesting because before we became a corporate entity, still small-town-culture oriented, I had much more to say about coming in during the middle of the night or other after-hours times. For example, I could decide to meet and treat someone who was having a COPD [chronic obstructive pulmonary disease] exacerbation or whatever might be an urgent situation and save that person 90-mile round-trip to the nearest ER. Occasionally, I might have the person come to my home and say, "I cut myself, can you sew me up?" and I would meet that person at the clinic. Now, it's a much more complicated process as the patient has to be registered into the EMR system so that you can bill for the service, but I have not been trained to register patients (and don't have the time) to do that. So now it's a matter of okay, if somebody calls me, yes I'll take care of him or her, but how do you get around this

whole electronic way of dealing with billing without causing a lot of extra work for the other office staff. They [corporate] don't want me to have to deal with things from home and I'm not sure what underlies that. Do they not want to pay for the time I spend doing that, or does it not fit into their model? This personal, availability of care is integral within the culture of frontier, which is another piece of what is not being considered in decision making, from a corporate-based model.

The on-call discussion brought up the issue of providing care to family and friends. Sue likes to keep her provider role separate from her friend or family role:

I do have a couple of very close, close friends and I've asked them not to see me as a regular provider. I'll take care of any urgent problems, but I'm too close to them and they've been very respectful of that.

Sue does feel that knowing all your patients on multiple levels and in different roles can be very advantageous:

I've had many patients who I've had to give really bad news to, but it's interesting because I feel like, I'm glad it's me. I can cry with them, I can see them through it.

Sue also says that her relationship with her community members changed when her role changed from clinic RN to clinic NP:

As I went into the NP role, it's isolated me more. A very interesting thing, I don't feel the same camaraderie I did as when I was the RN. It's really changed the dynamics of relationships and I'm not sure it's all related to becoming the NP. I'm not as active in the community now as when my kids were in school.

As her kids graduated, moved away, and started having families of their own, Sue's involvement in the community has lessened. In earlier days she added to the social capital in her community primarily through her professional role. She coordinated a health fair, lectured in the local high school science class, and was instrumental in bringing mobile mammography to this community. The mobile van now comes four times a year.

The issue of confidentiality is an aspect of frontier NP practice that is discussed in the literature:

People will stop me in the store, in front of other people and they start asking me questions. I've developed a really nice way of saying, "I want the best care for you and trying to take care of this here in the grocery store isn't going to give you the benefit of my attention and my best. So I need you to make an appointment." Once, I was checking out at the store and the cashier says, "You know, you know more about me than my husband," and I'm thinking, please don't tell me that in front of the 10 people in line. But it was funny and you know that's just part of it.

When asked what she thought would happen to the clinic, she had this to say:

I think that as long as there is some value here, financially as a rural clinic, and I don't know how to exactly quantify that, the clinic will survive. We don't provide ancillary services locally and send many people out of this community to get these services. So, even if it is not highly profitable in numbers of patients who walk through the door, there is profit from what is gained through federally funded rural programs or services, but I have a real question about that, because there isn't a lot of concern about finding out what the frontier culture consists of and how the optimal delivery of health care is different from the metropolitan areas.

And when asked about her plans, Sue said, "I hope to practice another 5 or 10 years, maybe more as I could see practicing until I'm 70, I still love it."

■ THEMES

Themes that emerged from Sue's story are: *go with the flow or swim against the current*, *frontier culture*, and *distance quarterbacking*. A subtheme of the first theme, go with the flow or swim against the current, is *change*. In this analysis the term *go with the flow* represents acceptance of, or adaptation to, change.

Sue uses the word "change" repeatedly throughout the interview. This begins when she talks about how her illness changed her career plans and her location. She had never planned to live in her current community, and in fact she had explicitly told her husband she wouldn't. Now she says that even if they move to be closer to their aging parents, they hope to always keep their current home. Change came again as the children entered school and she started to work 1 day a week at the clinic. This led to another change 10 years later when she entered an NP program. She then changed roles and when she had become comfortable in that position, the clinic changed ownership. The new corporate entity almost immediately began changing routines, providers, and technology at the clinic. It is evident in her story that Sue has adapted to change throughout her adult life and she has adapted to some of the clinic changes. She is able to see both the good and the bad that technological change has brought. She also sees the positive and negative impacts that an integrated system has brought to her patients, the community, and the clinic.

Sue's resistance to change is represented by the term *swim against the current*. This resistance to change was evident in Bob and Pam's narratives while Ann used political power to resist change. Their motivation to swim against the current, against the current of new health care policy, is to prevent the disintegration of the health care safety net in frontier America.

Sue also uses the term *frontier culture* throughout her narrative. She uses this term to denote a difference between the priorities of corporate America and those of frontier communities. Sue talks about the difference between the thought processes of corporate America and those of rural/ frontier America. This concept is related to Jim's explanation of the *different mindset*, which one needs to practice in these settings. It also relates to the insider–outsider concept, though, on a larger scale.

The theme distance quarterbacking emerged as Sue told the story of caring for the young female patient with several medical problems. It also emerged in another situation when Sue was trying to sort out a patient's multisystem complaint. She was not able to use her electronic system as she had with the first patient. This patient wanted his diagnostic tests done at a hospital more than 100 miles to the north:

> So we coordinated care via telephone rather than electronically and we set all of these appointments up for him. He was able to travel on one specific date because his wife can only take him on one day of the week. So, he ended up seeing the neurologist who wants to get an MRI of the brain because we've been thinking his problems may stem from his spine. So he wants that done, and a spinal tap. He's having this continual lower leg swelling so we're thinking we'd better check for a DVT [deep vein thrombosis] and

he wants it all done in one day. This is on a Friday, my day off, no one's in the clinic and they're trying to find me and tell me that he does have a DVT. He had left the ultrasound department and went to have the spinal tap. I'm trying to track him down because I'm in . . . on my day off, talking to the radiologist who's trying to let me know what's going on. I said you're going to have to try and find this guy [chuckling] he's up there somewhere in your hospital. By the time they track him down he's already had his last test and left. He doesn't have his cell phone turned on so we're trying to track him down through either a daughter or someone that might know where he's going next. Since this is a little town you know where everyone is going and when. So, we know the pharmacy he uses and we try to leave a message there to have him call us so we can get him started on Lovenox. He gets all the way home, he has been gone all day, gets back to our community and we don't have Lovenox here, in fact we don't have a pharmacy. So we sent him 55 miles south of here, to a rural ER so he could get the medication he needed. And this is all extra; this is all in an extra day of trying to coordinate care for a patient from a distance.

After listening to Sue's story one must ask oneself, if a rotating provider had gotten the call from the radiologist, would he or she have done as much to find this man? Would the radiologist even know where to start looking? The next question one has to ask oneself is, would the corporate entity even recognize and pay Sue for the amount of time and effort put into distance quarterbacking this one patient situation?

■ CONCLUSION

Sue's story gives us a glimpse into health care changes that are occurring across frontier America. The question is, can the health care delivery model change without compromising care in these communities? Sue's story also illustrates the outsider concept in regard to corporate America and a frontier culture. Lastly, Sue's story illustrates the continuity-of-care concept in frontier NP practice. The quarterbacking, or care coordination, provided by Sue without compensation, on her day off, from more than 100 miles away, exemplifies the professionalism and ethics of frontier NP practice.

9

Amy: A Mobile Experience

■ OVERVIEW

Amy's interview takes place in a frontier community clinic, after a long workday and long after the clinic staff have gone home. As is typical, she is alone in the clinic trying to finish up her work, returning patients' phone calls, checking lab results, and charting.

Amy is now the sole provider at the clinic, but this was not always the case. Amy had originally been hired to work on the mobile van. A few years earlier the clinic merged with a larger health care organization. Prior to the merge, the clinic had employed a part-time nurse practitioner (NP) to work on their mobile van. The mobile clinic had provided health care to a small community (basically a gas station/mini-mart and a post office) 20 miles away, but this service was terminated after the merge.

An opportunity to work on the mobile van came at a time when Amy and her husband were considering purchasing a home in the community. They had been vacationing in the area for more than 10 years and felt it was time to buy a second home. The part-time employment income would offset the cost of a second home and also allow her to spend more time in a community that she loved:

> I liked the idea of going out on the mobile clinic and taking care of the rural poor because that was the way I perceived the NP role. It was to take care of *all* people of all ages and financial statuses, and to take care of the rural poor.

Prior to enrolling in an NP program, Amy had been a surgical clinical nurse specialist (CNS) and assisted surgeons in the operating room:

> I built up the Medicare program for surgical assisting and because of the crossover with medical practice, the hospital wouldn't allow me to do it while I was on duty as an

RN. I had to take the extra step of clocking out and being *independent* when I was in that role. Some of the surgeons also wanted me to work in their offices but as a CNS I couldn't get prescriptive authority, so I needed to get an NP license. The *carrot* for the NP role was the independent piece that the NP role was supposed to be an autonomous and independent role for nurses.

Prior to entering into frontier practice, Amy's emergency care experiences were limited. Besides her CNS experience in the operating room, she had telemetry and cardiac catheter lab experience. She honed her suturing skills by assisting with surgical cases and eventually taught a suturing class for NP students.

■ CONCEPTS

The concept of the frontier NP as an expert generalist and multitasker was discussed in the literature review. Amy's prior experiences proved helpful when faced with situations that involved this concept:

> I was on the mobile clinic and a man came in who was having an MI [myocardial infarction]. When he walked onto the van he had no blood pressure, he had no chest pain. So you do the EKG and you see that he's having an MI and you call for a helicopter. The problem with the little town we were parked in was they didn't have an ambulance, they had a rescue truck. So it's either put him on the back of a flat-bed rescue truck, or drive him to the landing zone in the mobile van. So, I've got a patient in the back of the van, I'm holding onto him while the driver is driving. I had the IV in him, I had him all packaged and ready to go. So, you have to be able to multitask. You have to start an IV, put him on oxygen, and give medications without the help of backup, you're doing it all yourself.

Sometimes, a receiving trauma center can make assumptions about the level of care that can reasonably be provided in a frontier setting without delaying transport of a critically injured patient:

> The river was extraordinarily high one year and a tourist jumped into the river for a swim, hit his head on a rock and

nearly de-scalped himself. He was hemorrhaging by the time the volunteers were called and the ambulance got him to the clinic, he was losing his blood pressure. I didn't even have time to give him local anesthesia, I had to say, "I'm sorry sir, but if I don't do this you may die." I managed to slow down the bleeding by rapidly closing the wound with staples before he was flown to the trauma center (120 miles away). I called the trauma center a couple hours later to see how he was doing, "Oh, that guy's doing great. We're getting ready to send him home." I asked if they had explored his wound and they replied no. So I said, I think you better because there could be pebbles in his head, all I did was close his wound because he was bleeding to death!

Another concept identified in the literature review is the need to handle multiple trauma or emergent patient situations with few resources:

That's hard. I had a situation like that last summer. There was a lady at one of the local businesses and she looked like she was coding. We get her to the clinic, do an EKG and she's got ischemic changes. Miraculously she woke up, but before we could provide further treatment, there's another call. There's been a head-on collision down the road. The gurney that the MI patient was on was the only gurney that the fire department had because the other ambulance was out of service. So I have potentially three victims with one ambulance, one gurney, and one provider!

Besides a lack of emergency medical services (EMS) and mental health services, frontier communities often lack hospice services. Amy and the clinic provide much of this service by prescribing medications and making frequent home visits to monitor the patient and support the families. Even with this support, sometimes families bring their loved ones to the clinic near the end:

The clinic is a place to come for urgent care, emergencies, and routine care. It is also a place for somebody to come when they're in pain and when they're dying. With one particular terminal patient, her daughter called me at a quarter to six in the morning and said something's going on with mom . . . and so basically we bring mom to the clinic where she dies. So that's all part of the frontier practice. I'm sure babies are born in the frontier too. But people also come to clinic because they're in severe pain, they come here to die or the family chooses their loved one to stay at home and we support them. It's good up until the end but then sometimes they need the comfort and support of the clinic.

The concept of a rural skillset was discussed in the literature review. Some participants in this inquiry have discussed additional skills or capabilities that are necessary for frontier NP practice. When asked about the concept of a rural skillset, Amy had this to say:

> If you can make decisions and if you can make the right decisions, you'll be successful. A lot of nurses in my NP program were smart, but if you're not able to make a decision on your own, you're not going to be successful. I think that's the hardest part of being an NP in a frontier area, you might find some backup but you might *not* find backup, you're pretty much on your own.

Near the end of the interview I asked Amy if she had anything more she wanted to say. Her answer highlights the holistic nature of frontier NP practice:

> I'm not sure where the role is going at this point in time. I think frontier medicine is the way medicine used to be practiced in this country, taking care of the person from birth through the life cycle until death. The old-time doctor used to do home visits, would be called out at all hours of the night to see his patients, but that type of medicine has changed. I mean you can't afford to have a doctor in a frontier area and that's truly the role of the NP. Besides the medical piece of frontier NP practice there's also the nursing piece of being able to start IVs, do wound care, dressing changes, all the things that nurses do. Like, put a Foley catheter in for someone who can't urinate. I think doctors are better at giving directions or orders; where I think the frontier NP role is more of a hands-on role, it's a combination of medicine and nursing.

As a result of a corporate decision, Amy's clinic recently stopped providing 24/7 care. Now, after-hours calls are answered by a service located in a larger community. The clinic NP no longer has the ability to triage the calls and there is no advanced cardiac life support available on evenings or weekends when the clinic is closed:

> I'm kind of concerned about the future of health care in frontier areas because healthcare is changing, it's more automated. We have the electronic record, we're going more to free-standing clinics that are open nine to five, there's nobody available in the evening to talk to. Patients are directed by someone on the answering service who directs them to go to the emergency room. Then we have the problem with the overflow of the emergency room.

Amy continues with a statement that illustrates frontier NP ethics: "We're always going to have rural and frontier areas in America, and we're always going to have the rural poor, and we have an obligation to make sure everyone gets care."

◼ THEMES

Two themes emerge from Amy's narrative that relate to frontier NP practice: *independence* and *cradle to grave*. The theme independence was evident from the first story segment, where she states that it was the independent and autonomous role of the NP that motivated her to enroll in an NP program. She provides examples of *doing it yourself* or *you're on your own*, and *making your own decisions*, throughout her story segments. She also states, "I don't think in urban America the NP role is such an independent and autonomous role, you have to look at rural and frontier areas to see the practice in the way that the NP role was intended."

The theme, cradle to grave care, is a concept alluded to when Amy describes the range of care provided by frontier NPs (from birth to death). This phrase can also connote holistic care, the type of care that Amy described when asked what she wanted readers to know about frontier practice. Amy also states that people of all ages and financial statuses should have access to health care. All participants in this study were family NPs. This indicates that they have been educated to provide care to patients across the life cycle. This is also representative of cradle to grave care, which is what NPs who practice in a community setting must provide.

■ CONCLUSION

Amy started her NP career in the back of a mobile van. When a corporate merge threatened to leave the clinic with only rotating physicians, unfamiliar with the clinic and the townspeople, Amy stepped in and agreed to be the solo NP. She said the town deserved to have a medical clinic and she would do the best she could to help keep it open. Amy's ethics and dedication to her community are evident in both her words and her actions.

10

Lori: A Career Choice

■ OVERVIEW

Lori left frontier nurse practitioner (NP) practice several years ago due to unforeseen family issues. She spent a total of 17 years in frontier NP practice; two of these were during her NP training. Lori was working as an acute care medical–surgical nurse in a rural hospital prior to applying to an NP program. She had planned on pursuing a master's degree in nursing education but was unsure if she wanted to leave direct patient care. While working at the hospital, "I met a nurse who lived in a frontier community about an hour away. She worked part time at the hospital and part time as a home-health nurse for a rural health clinic in her frontier community." Lori was intrigued with this notion of a *frontier* practice and eventually learned that the clinic director was an NP. "I drove up to meet this frontier NP and was amazed at the variety of patients and problems that were seen there and the complexity of care that the remote clinic offered. Right then and there I made the choice to apply to NP school."

The clinic director agreed to precept Lori and she spent the majority of her 2-year training program at the frontier clinic. She was hired 2 weeks after graduation: "My preceptor, and now clinic partner, left for his yearly vacation two weeks after I was hired. I was on my own with a summertime population that was easily 10 times that of the year round population." Lori and her partner split 24/7 call, but with her colleague on vacation she covered call five out of seven nights with a locum tenens physician covering the weekends. This went on for a month: "It was kind of trial by fire; my clinic RN would come to me and say, 'the waiting room is getting pretty full,' while I was rummaging through texts trying to get my diagnosis and treatment plan correct." Even though she had a rough start, "I loved every minute of frontier practice. I loved taking care of people of all ages; I loved the wide range of problems, from well-care to emergent care." Lori states that one of the biggest benefits of frontier practice is really getting to know your patients and their families: "Case management is a big issue now a days, for us it was just the way things were done. We knew the patients, their families, and what their resources were. This was very helpful when you're dealing with a complex medical issue."

■ CONCEPTS

Lori took call as a routine aspect of her NP practice. A review of the literature indicates that being on call can cause personal challenges for a frontier NP:

> . . . yes, it's a challenge. In the summer you can be up half the night but still have to show up on time in the morning prepared for whatever comes through the front door. Since there were only two of us to cover a call schedule we overlapped just one day per week. If the waiting room was still full at 5 o'clock, there was no point in going home because if you were the one on call that night, you'd just be right back. We provided medical coverage for the jail and on the weekend you could almost guarantee a call out at 2 a.m. to draw blood for a potential DUI [driving under the influence].

This last statement brought up the concept of role diffusion:

> You do everything because there's no one else to do it. The jail does not have a nurse to draw blood in the middle of the night, there's not enough inmates to justify that expense. The county doesn't always have a coroner on duty either. I've had to pronounce kayakers and rafters on the side of the road after they've been pulled from the river. If you're on call during the weekend and the snow is covering the walkway to the clinic, you go shovel it. If someone needs blood drawn, you're a phlebotomist; if they need an x-ray, you're the x-ray technician. I've even helped the sheriff's department in determining if skeletal remains were human or animal. I was shown the skeletal remains of a foot once and I honestly couldn't determine if it was human, or more likely, bear. I called a local retired vet and he explained that there was only a slight difference in lengths of one toe. I was

able to determine that it was, in fact, a bear's skeleton. Also, there is no local veterinarian but we do have a traveling vet who comes to town a couple of times a month. That's not much of a help the rest of the time. We have a lot of mining claims up here and people will leave rat bait out over the winter. Sure enough, first time they visit the claim in the summer they usually have a dog with them. Invariably the dog eats the rat bait. I've injected several dogs with vitamin K over the years. I've also treated dogs for rattlesnake bites with steroids to decrease the swelling . . . but that's one of the things I love about frontier practice, it's always different and you learn so much as a result.

In the literature review, Connor (2002) stated that knowledge of referral specialists is very helpful. Lori had mentioned use of a retired vet as a resource, so I asked if she used this type of informal referral source regularly:

Since we don't have any specialists up here it's really helpful to know who you *can* call. I remember one summer when a group of school kids went up to one of the local lakes on a swim trip. The following week I started to see kids in the clinic with an atypical rash. They appeared to have all been exposed to something at the lake. I finally called the county health director (he doesn't live in our county but he's in an adjacent county) and he told me it was probably just swimmer's itch. I spoke with one of the old-timers about it and he said, "Yes, everybody knows to stay away from that lake right after the duck migration or you get a rash." Chalk one up for local knowledge, I could have saved a lot of time by just asking him first [chuckles]. It was also good to know the ER [emergency room] physicians at the local hospital [a rural hospital 55 miles away]. They are a good resource if you're unsure about something, like maybe a minor EKG abnormality that you're not sure you should send. Also, if you build a good rapport with them they develop trust in your judgment. For example, if you have a trauma but you think the local hospital can handle it, they are more likely to accept the transfer based on your judgment. This is important for patients because if you send them to a trauma hospital and they're discharged later that day, their family has to drive an additional 1 to 2 hours to pick them up. Some of my patients just didn't have the resources to cover that kind of travel.

The provision of emergency medical and trauma care has been noted to be one of the biggest differences between rural and frontier nursing. I asked Lori about her experiences with this:

The first time I met with the clinic director to discuss precepting at his clinic he told me I needed some ER experience. I was just finishing my BSN program at the time [Lori had been an RN for 8 years] and still hadn't chosen an area of concentration for my advanced nursing course. So before I started the NP program I used the opportunity to work in a fairly busy ER for a semester. Certifications in ACLS [advanced cardiac life support] and PALS [pediatric advanced life support] were required to work at the clinic and I eventually got my MICN [mobile intensive care nurse] certification that allowed me to direct the volunteer ambulance crew. The locals only had BLS [basic life support] certifications, which meant the clinic NPs were the most qualified people to provide emergency and trauma care. That didn't mean I was comfortable with it, I never did get comfortable, but when someone's in trouble and you're the only one who has the knowledge to help, you do the best you can.

The provision of medical care to family and friends has also been discussed in the literature. When asked about this concept, Lori told this story:

Since I was the only female provider at the clinic I did most of the Ps [Pap smears] which included a lot of first-time Paps for girls. I tried to make it as nonthreatening as possible. I would show them all the equipment ahead of time, including the *salad spoons*, or speculum, and we would get a pretty good laugh out of it. Many times it was a family affair with mom there too. I'm a big talker and since I knew the girls and their families, I could usually come up with a conversation that would distract them during the procedure. Even so, more than once, after I was done, the girl would look at me and say, "I won't be able to look at you on the street now because I'm embarrassed." I would always say, don't worry, for me it's just like looking at your tonsils, but I understand. Even though the girls said that, it never happened, they were always okay with it.

Lori goes on to say this about privacy and the Health Insurance Portability and Accountability Act (HIPAA) when providing family planning services in a frontier community:

> I had known many of these girls, and boys, since they were little. They knew me, they developed trust in me, so privacy was never really an issue. I would tell the kids that if they ever needed to see me about this and didn't want anyone to know, they could schedule an appointment for a fictitious reason (so they didn't have to worry about the receptionist knowing) and we would deal with it in the privacy of the exam room. By the time I started working at the clinic people were a lot more open about these sort of things. However, my clinic partner had prescribed birth control pills to a girl a few years before and her dad found out about it and showed up at the clinic very angry. I would always encourage my younger patients to tell their parents if they were seeking family planning services but I never made them feel like they *had* to.

Lori also had this to say about what it was like to work in the frontier:

> I love the close-knit nature of a frontier community. Even though every one knows everyone else's business, it's still nice to know that people have one another's backs. There was an older couple that lived on Main Street, right next to the diner. The husband didn't drive any more, but the wife did. One day she was driving to the next town and got in a minor car accident. She was transported to a hospital, about an hour away, just for observation overnight. The next morning I was running into the diner before work when I saw a sign in the window of Mr. X's house that read, HELP I need coffee. Within an hour he had more coffee and food than he knew what to do with. This probably would have never happened in a larger town. When you get to know people, you just naturally want to help them. I used to walk my dog every night. There were three bridges across the river that ran through town

so there were three possible loops that you could walk. Without stopping I could make the middle loop in about 25 minutes. It always took me an hour because you would stop to talk to different neighbors along the way. It really made me feel connected to the community. Also, our town was too remote to have mail delivery to your doorstep so everyone used the post office. If someone were born, someone died, or anything interesting was happening in town, it was posted on the post office door. I never felt out of touch while I lived there.

When asked if there was anything else Lori wanted to add, she had this to say:

Although I loved working in the frontier I don't want people to think it was all rosy. The call-time places a strain on personal and family life. There were many times I felt stretched beyond my capacity; either there wasn't enough of me to go around or I felt I was in a situation that was over my head. You are presented with so many different problems in the frontier, there is no way you can be prepared for all of it. You need to know your resources and how to find answers for the unusual cases. I had a huge wilderness medicine book on my office shelf, I didn't use it much but when I needed it, it was there. I dealt with raccoon, ferret, snake, and scorpion bites. I also dealt with a couple of cases of altitude sickness. I had the CDC [Centers for Disease Control and Prevention] website book-marked. You might think that living in an isolated area you are protected from emerging diseases but during the SARS [severe acute respiratory syndrome] outbreak in the 90s we had a local couple who had returned from China, they had been there during the outbreak. Also, back when H1N1 was first recognized as a threat in this country, I diagnosed the first case in our county. Our county public health agency was on the other side of a mountain pass, so on our side of the county we did a lot of public health surveillance. This included TB [tuberculosis] surveillance. I was the first provider to order a Quantiferon Gold test for an equivocal PPD [purified protein derivative] reading. So just because you're remote, you still need to be up on current health issues.

Lori had this final comment:

The hours are long and the pay is less than most RNs make in acute care but the experience was invaluable. I had patients who will be lifelong friends and you can never have too many of those. But the most important thing is that I felt like I was making a difference in people's lives and generally improving the health of the community. So in the balance, I feel like I gained much more than I gave.

▓ THEMES

Several previously identified themes are evident in Lori's narrative. Lori's statements about the many roles she assumed in her practice fits under the theme of *many hats*. This was not only evident during normal clinic hours when other staff is present, but even more evident when she was the only provider during off hours. These roles were not only task oriented, such as phlebotomy and x-ray, but represented different roles such as MICN and public health officer. *Flying solo* was also evident in Lori's narrative when she discussed being the only provider on call and not having specialty backup in her community. *Cradle to grave* was represented by Lori's statements regarding caring for people of all ages. The concept of insider/outsider falls under the theme of *frontier culture*. In the literature, the idea of being an outsider can be a barrier to frontier practice; however, Lori foresaw this issue and took specific measures to overcome it. The theme of being *out on a limb* was represented by Lori's statement that sometimes she felt she was in situations that were over her head.

Leadership has been a recurring theme with all the narratives. Lori talked about joining the board of directors and volunteering for hiring committees for local government agencies. These activities demonstrate community leadership. Lori also volunteered to provide transportation for the local schoolkids to out-of-town games. These are both examples of how NPs add to the *social capital* of frontier communities.

Several additional themes are evident in Lori's narrative. The first is the *connectivity* she felt with not only her patients, but the community in general. When asked what it was like to practice in a frontier area, Lori's first response was a story about the close-knit nature of frontier communities. Lori states that "knowing everyone's business" has positive and negative repercussions:

Sometimes it's hard for patients and their families to separate your personal and professional roles. Being someone's friend outside the clinic can make it hard to say no when it comes to prescribing things like pain medication. On the other hand, being friends with a patient can help if you have to give them bad news. A patient, and husband of one of my close friends, had recently been diagnosed with malignant melanoma. He was being monitored by a specialist at a tertiary care center. He came to the clinic because he noticed another mole that he thought didn't look right. We excised it and the biopsy came back positive for another melanoma. I knew my friend and her husband would be really upset about this because the implications of two malignancies aren't good. I called them up and asked if I could come by their house during my lunch break. They knew I was at work and they were waiting for the result. I wanted to give them time to mentally prepare for the information. When I got to their house we sat on the front porch, in rocking chairs, and calmly discussed the biopsy results. I think that receiving the results in the environment of their own home made it less scary for them and they were able to absorb the information and make plans calmly.

The second is *lifelong learning*. The need to promote this competency in nursing has been promoted by Benner, Sutphen, Leonard, and Day (2010) and others and is crucial when working in an environment where there is no one to turn to for answers but yourself. Lori expressed this theme when discussing having Internet and print resources as well as human resources to call upon. It was also evident when Lori was discussing emerging diseases.

The third is *interdisciplinary practice*. Lori felt she worked cooperatively with the sheriff's department, the volunteer fire department/ambulance crew, and the county health department.

We kept a full range of medications at the clinic, including opiates. If I got called to the clinic, late at night, for a patient that I didn't know, I would always call the sheriff's department (their office was across the street from the clinic) and I would tell them that I was going to leave the ER door open and to please keep an eye out for me. They always did. Also, if I had an after-hours emergency at the clinic and I thought I needed help, I knew I could always call on the fire department volunteers and they would come right over. This wasn't a one-sided relationship, I was just as willing to help these departments as they were to help me.

Lori goes on to say:

The nature of my practice meant that I was closer to the fire department. They were volunteers of all ages, gender, and skill level. They didn't have the fanciest equipment but they knew how to make do and use what they had. Sometimes when they transported patients to the hospital down the hill, the professionals would sometimes treat them as country boys or girls, like they weren't as good as the paid crews. I really took offense to this; I was, and still am, very proud of the selfless work they did. They worked for the good of the community and gave it *their all*, many times risking life and limb to help others. My colleague and I would conduct training classes for them and in return, we would attend their run reviews. Many times we would attend training sessions provided by outside agencies that the fire department brought in. I remember attending a cold-water drowning class in the community hall that was very informative and impacted my practice. We just called it working together, and now they call it interdisciplinary practice [laughs].

The *ethics* of frontier practice reveal themselves in Lori's narrative, particularly when she discusses building trust with the local ER physicians so that her patients and their families wouldn't incur hardships by traveling to a hospital farther away. The ethical concept of *duty* is evident in Lori's narrative as she shared another story involving frontier practice:

I was on call one evening when I received a call from the hospital ER. The ER physician had been alerted by the lab regarding a critical INR [international normalized ratio]. Earlier in the day we sent down an INR on a patient who was taking Coumadin. The INR was critically elevated at more than nine and they lived 15 miles up the hill. The ER physician asked me if I was planning to send the patient to the ER for treatment to lower the INR. I told him that I would be worried about the patient's travelling either

15 miles to the clinic or 70 miles to the hospital, possibly getting into an accident and bleeding out. I told the ER physician that I would drive to the patient's house and give them an injection of vitamin K and some oral vitamin K tabs to take over the next few days. He replied that he had never heard of a provider doing something like that for a patient. I told him that I felt it was my duty to make sure the patient was safe.

Ethical comportment was also evident when Lori walked to her patient's house to "give him the news" about his biopsy results; it is also an example of the *caring* that is evident in Lori's practice.

■ CONCLUSION

Lori's narrative supported many of the themes that are common to other participants. NPs who practice and live in frontier communities become *embedded* in those communities. It becomes difficult to separate out the role of NP from the role of community member. This promotes leadership, caring, and, from the evidence in the narratives, ethical comportment.

REFERENCES

Benner, P., Sutphen, M., Leonard, V., & Day, L. (2010). *Educating nurses: A call for radical transformation*. San Francisco, CA: Jossey-Bass.

Connor, M. (2002). Transitioning to rural primary care. *Advance for Nurse Practitioners, 10*(6), 83–84.

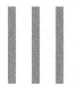

The Model

Part III introduces the conceptual model for frontier nurse practitioner (NP) practice. The foundation of the model is the narrative nursing knowledge revealed in the participant narratives. Narrative knowledge is based on nursing experience, and its contribution to nursing practice is well established.

Nursing practice changes over time. It is influenced by scientific advances, evidence-based research, and technology. As nursing models are a guide for practice, they cannot be static; they must be flexible enough to withstand the test of time. The four types of knowledge that support effective NP practice are broad enough to encompass the advances that will inevitably occur.

The conceptual model for frontier NP practice is a guide for practice, education, research, and policy. Examples of utilization of the model in all of these areas are provided. The participants in this book are passionate about frontier health care and want their experiences to both guide others and affect health care policy. Part III concludes with recommendations in three areas: educational preparation for frontier NP practice, frontier research, and frontier health care policy.

11

Narrative Knowledge

The concepts related to frontier nurse practitioner (NP) practice noted in the Chapter 3 summary of the literature (Table 3.1) are supported by the participant narratives. Additional concepts and themes emerged from the participant stories. These concepts, and the themes that exemplify them, represent *narrative knowledge*. This chapter illustrates how this narrative knowledge was utilized to support a conceptual model for frontier NP practice.

■ REFLECTED EXPERIENCE AS KNOWLEDGE

Experiences have both an interior and an exterior landscape (Gadow, 1995). The interior landscape represents introspection, when one examines one's own thoughts or feelings related to an experience; in contrast, the exterior landscape represents the facts related to the experience. Narratives present a holistic view of experience as they combine both landscapes simultaneously. This allows the narrator to simultaneously relate a chronology of events while critically reflecting on those events.

When nurses relate stories of nursing situations, the stories represent *reflected* experience. The reflected experience is not identical to the experience itself; it occurs only in retrospect when the worth of the meanings, or cognitive ideas, is critically inspected in view of the results of the experience (Dewey, 1969–1991, pp. 27–28). Reflected experience, as knowledge, exists within nursing actions in an implicit and uniquely personal fashion. This occurs because reflected knowledge is derived from experiences that are inherently unique and value laden (Medina & Castillo, 2006). When reflected experience is expressed in story form, the reflected knowledge becomes narrative knowledge.

Narratives allow nurses to communicate nursing praxis. This occurs because narratives reveal the entirety of the nursing situation. *Praxis* is a term that connotes value-grounded, thoughtful reflection and action that occur in synchrony (Chinn & Kramer, 1999, p. 256). Narratives include not only the events and outcomes, but also the narrator's feelings and the thought processes utilized during the situation. This is much different than observing a nursing situation; it is enhanced by reflection of the narrator. Narrative knowledge results from this reflection; it is the synchrony of the cognitive, the aesthetic, and the moral knowing (Nairn, 2004). It is through this mechanism that the stories in this book represent narrative knowledge regarding frontier NP practice.

■ TYPES OF FRONTIER KNOWLEDGE

Nurses care for patients in a holistic manner. This requires different types of knowledge that synchronize to inform nursing actions. The narrative knowledge illustrated in the participant stories synchronizes several types of knowledge, or *ways of knowing*.

In 1978, Barbara Carper introduced four patterns, or ways of knowing, nursing knowledge: (a) empirical, (b) esthetics, (c) personal knowledge, and (d) ethics. Peggy Chinn and Maeona Kramer (1999) advanced Carper's theory by proposing that these knowledge patterns originate from one of four knowledge domains: (a) empirics, or scientific competence; (b) personal, the therapeutic use of self; (c) ethics, the moral/ethical comportment of nursing practice; and (d) aesthetics; transformative nursing art/acts. They further theorized that these knowledge domains do not stand alone; rather, each domain informs and is informed by the others. Sally Gadow (1995, p. 213) contributed to the epistemological discussion by stating that narratives themselves are a way of knowing because through nursing stories we offer one another our experience.

Jill White (1995) proposed a fifth way of knowing: sociopolitical. Sociopolitical knowing addresses the *wherein* of nursing. It causes nurses to question the taken-for-granted assumptions about practice, the profession, and health policies. Sociopolitical knowing has two components: the sociopolitical context of the persons (nurse and patient), and the sociopolitical context of nursing as a practice profession. The second component includes both society's understanding of nursing and nursing's understanding of society and its politics.

The narrative knowledge revealed in the participant stories also follows patterns: (a) knowledge of skills that are distinct to frontier NP practice, (b) knowledge that is unique to the frontier context, (c) the political knowledge to make an impact in frontier health care, and (d) art and ethics that are distinctly frontier oriented. It is the contention of this book that these four types of knowledge are required for effective frontier

NP practice, or praxis. The model depicts these types of knowledge as: (a) *contextual knowledge*, (b) *frontier skills and competencies*, (c) *political knowledge*, and (d) *art and ethics*. These four types of knowledge are discussed in the following sections.

Contextual Knowledge

Frontier NP practice is a specialty practice. Contextual knowledge is knowledge that is required for each type of specialty practice. This includes knowledge related to the concepts outlined in rural nursing theory. When taken to the frontier, these concepts have expanded meanings.

In rural nursing theory, health is primarily defined as the ability to work or be productive. Ann's narrative, which includes the story about the man who broke his leg but did not come into the clinic until the work was done, exemplifies this concept of rural nursing theory. When taken into the frontier, this definition of health also has *systems* implications. The notion that rural dwellers *don't stop working until the job is done* impacts the availability of volunteer emergency medical services (EMS) in frontier areas. Ann's narrative provides an example of this concept when she discusses the lack of volunteer EMS personnel during haying or harvesting season.

The notion that rural residents are self-reliant is evident throughout the narratives. In the frontier setting the adage *necessity is the mother of invention* is applicable. This self-reliance is primarily due to the lack of available resources. Ann's narrative exemplifies this notion when she discusses using farm gear in lieu of personal protective equipment. An entire community can also be self-reliant. As federal subsidies in frontier areas dwindle, frontier communities have turned inward for solutions to finance health care clinics in these areas. Ann's narrative is an example of this concept as her community developed its own local tax base to fund their health care needs.

In rural nursing theory, the concept of insider/outsider is related both to the skepticism that rural dwellers have about accepting help or services from outsiders, and to the notion that health care providers who are new to the community are outsiders. Bob describes his first day of frontier NP practice, a day when he went above and beyond the community's expectations of a health care provider. Bob felt this gave him credibility with the community. This implies that as a newcomer he needed to gain acceptance. This supports Long and Weinert's statement that some nurses use community involvement to gain acceptance. Community involvement is related to the idea of social capital, which is a concept woven through the narratives.

Skepticism about accepting help or services from outsiders was supported by the narratives as well. Bob states that receiving the 330 grant was both a "godsend and a curse." Most participants relied on grant funding and federal programs to prop up frontier health care systems; however, they are worried about changes in federal priorities that could dry up these funding sources.

In this book, the concept of outsider also applies to a broader context, the perspective that federal or corporate agencies have regarding health care in the frontier. Outsiders try to "put a round peg in a square hole" when it comes to policies regarding the provision of health care and related services in frontier areas. This concept was exemplified by one of the themes that emerged from Ann's story: *it doesn't work here.*

Role diffusion has been described as the need to function in multiple roles both in one's personal and professional life (Long & Weinert, 1989). For a rural nurse, this might mean working across several hospital departments in one shift. The examples provided by Long and Weinert were: (a) doing an EKG, (b) drawing labs, (c) delivering babies, or (d) cooking meals if the hospital was snowed in. In the frontier, this concept is extended to include skillsets beyond patient care. Both Bob and Ann discussed the need to act as both the clinic administrator and the clinic provider. Bob exemplified this concept when he discussed the need to build reimbursement systems for his clinic and the need to write grants to maintain services. Lori also exemplified the concept of role diffusion when she talked about shoveling snow on the walkway into the clinic.

The concept of lack of anonymity is widely supported in the narratives. This is exemplified with the concept of *reciprocity of care,* a theme that emerged from Pam's narrative. This concept was reinforced by Lori, who stated, "Everyone knows everyone else's business." It was also exemplified by Pam, who chuckled at the thought of privacy in a small town and stated that everyone knew whose car was parked in front of the clinic.

The themes *frontier culture, a different mindset, a barren health care landscape, it doesn't work here,* and *flying solo* all support the concept of contextual knowledge related to frontier NP practice. To practice effectively, frontier NPs must have knowledge regarding frontier culture. This includes specific knowledge related to local industries and economies. This may also include knowledge about seasonal practices such as harvesting and haying, which may affect local resources. This is knowledge very similar to that which is required for industrial nursing. Frontier NPs must familiarize themselves with treatment for the common injuries in their geographic setting. This may include injuries related to farm equipment, logging, or mining. In recreational areas, this may extend to knowledge regarding bicycle, motorcycle, snowmobile, or skiing injuries.

To practice effectively in frontier settings, NPs must have a different mindset. NPs must have knowledge of both formal and informal local resources. They must keep in mind that frontier dwellers live in a barren health care landscape and have limited health care resources. Referrals for specialty care or sophisticated diagnostics may have to be reserved for complex or unusual cases. It doesn't work here means that to practice effectively, frontier NPs need to know what *does* work in their clinic or their community. It may require adaptation of practices learned either in their NP programs, or from prior work experiences. It may also involve using knowledge and skill to bring new systems—systems that *do* work in the frontier setting. This implies knowledge of what is needed and how to get it accomplished, such as grant writing or the use of innovative technology.

Skills and Competencies

The concept of the frontier NP as an expert generalist is well documented. The narratives in this book demonstrate the wide range of skills that frontier NPs utilize. The participants managed situations ranging from emergency/trauma care to caring for pets and identifying skeletal remains. This wide skillset also encompasses the care of patients across the life span, from the cradle to the grave.

Flying by the seat of your pants implies being in a situation where either there are no protocols to follow or little is known about the situation. This requires a wide array of clinical skills and knowledge to proceed in an ethical manner. It may also involve writing new protocols, ones that reflect the available resources and referral networks.

Both specialty care and the availability of specialized diagnostic equipment are severely lacking in frontier communities. Gary Lausten's (2013) study demonstrated that rural NPs utilized a wider variety of procedures than urban NPs. In the frontier, competency involves not only the ability to perform procedures, but the ability to practice in isolated settings with limited resources. Therefore, to accurately diagnose patients' problems, frontier NPs primarily rely on their history taking and clinical exam skills. This involves both maintaining a current knowledge base and the use of available resources to find answers to patient problems.

In situations when a patient must be sent to a larger service area for diagnostics or referrals, the NP may have to act as a *distance quarterback* to provide patient-centered coordination of care.

To practice effectively in frontier settings, NPs must be capable of flying solo; that is, practicing *independently*. As solo providers, frontier NPs must be capable of providing comprehensive primary care, including managing emergency/trauma situations and mental health concerns. At times these situations may involve more than one patient. This requires strong organizational skills and the ability to make quick decisions in emergent situations.

The ability to take and read x-rays has been identified as an important frontier skill. This ability enhances both diagnostic and triage capabilities in the frontier. Sending patients to the nearest hospital to have a chest or extremity x-ray might not be a reasonable choice, as some patients lack private transportation. Removing an EMS ambulance from the community for up to 6 hours due to an avoidable emergency department (ED) transport could prove fatal to the next emergency patient.

Mental health resources are severely lacking in frontier communities. Five of the seven participants found this lack of services to be particularly challenging. Ann felt that even one untreated patient caused significant financial hardship for her community. The case she cited also caused extreme stress on the local resources.

In Chapter 2, it was noted that teen suicide is higher in frontier areas. Jim's narrative illustrates how one frontier NP can make a difference. The narratives illustrate that frontier NPs must be comfortable prescribing medications used to treat common mental health conditions and they must also have a working knowledge of the regional referral system for acute cases. Additionally, NPs use their social capital to promote informal mental health services such as support groups and crisis interventions.

Interdisciplinary practice was evident in the exemplars. Ann stated that she "couldn't sustain a life" without the emergency medical technicians (EMTs); Lori depended on and worked closely with both the fire department and the sheriff's department; and Bob, Lori, and Ann had all trained emergency services volunteers. The narratives indicate that these working relationships may have been initiated by the isolation that characterizes frontier communities; however, the narratives also indicate genuine mutual respect between the disciplines. This is illustrated by the exemplars, "we work together for the benefit of the patient," and "I really respect them for their selfless service."

Innovation is required in emergency situations and everyday practice. There are several examples of the use of innovation within the narratives.

Sue talks about the usefulness of the electronic medical record when consulting with specialty physicians. Pam talks about technology in the emergency room that allowed her to speak with off-site physicians during emergency situations. Ann wrote a thesis about the use of broadband for tele-health, and Bob wrote grants to get updated equipment, such as digital x-ray, for his community.

Political Knowledge

Political knowledge has two aspects: knowledge of policy and the knowledge of what is required to act or advocate for one's community. It is the knowledge of policy that is necessary for administration of a frontier clinic. There are multiple federal programs that support rural health clinics. Administrative and political knowledge are used reciprocally to help NPs stabilize access to local health care. The participant narratives provide evidence that frontier NPs utilize knowledge regarding funding sources, such as grants and programs that offer enhanced reimbursement rates, to benefit their communities. Although only two of the participants had administrative roles in their clinics, all participants were aware of specialized billing methods and enhanced reimbursement rates for rural services.

The theme *shifting sands* reflects changes in federal programs and policies regarding frontier health care. Soon after the first NPs graduated, federally subsidized physician extender programs were developed to assess the effectiveness of putting NPs and physician assistants (PAs) in rural areas. Partnering NPs with physician collaborators also provided a mechanism that allowed Medicare for pay for NP services. In 1977, enactment of the Rural Health Clinic Act further bolstered NP practice in rural and frontier areas. These programs were developed to ensure a Medicare safety net for the rural elderly, and to support existing rural and frontier health care systems, such as National Health Service Corps clinics. However, a shift occurred in the early 1990s, starting with the Federally Qualified Health Clinic (FQHC) program and culminating with the Affordable Care Act (ACA). These programs have shifted federal funding from programs that are geographically based to those that are population based, thereby leaving the future of frontier health care undecided. Effective frontier NPs keep abreast of health care policy and how changes impact health care in their communities.

Changes in policy have caused some frontier clinics to merge with larger health care organizations. These changes present both personal and professional challenges to NPs who provide care in these settings. NPs will need to decide when it is best to go with the flow, and work within new programs, and when to swim against the current, to muster both personal and political power to advocate for their communities through policy change.

Nurses advocate for health care equity among groups and ensure that the voices of the disenfranchised are heard. Advocating for the good of others involves leadership skills. It was evident throughout the narratives that the participants demonstrated leadership in their communities.

Art and Ethics

The art and ethics of nursing practice are intrinsically woven. Ethical knowledge guides behavior; it allows nurses to decide the best course of action in certain situations. The *art* of nursing entails how those ethical decisions are carried out. Both concepts are brought to light within the narratives.

Ethics can be conceived of as a personal/professional concept or more globally in terms of social justice. Woven throughout the narratives are examples of patient-centered, ethical situations. Some of the participants told stories about emergency situations, situations in which they felt *out on a limb* or *in over their heads.* These NPs had to make split-second decisions about the ethics of providing care. One might say that certain situations, such as delivering a double footling breech in a remote area, were beyond the scope and comfort of the NP involved. One option might have been to put the patient in an ambulance and hope she made it to the nearest obstetrician, 55 miles away. To quickly review your options, and decide to *buck up* and do the best you can, is an ethical one.

The same situation applies in Amy's case when she had to staple a patient's scalp without anesthesia. Before proceeding, she quickly explained the situation and gave the patient the option to say no. Not exploring the wound first was an understandable breach in care; therefore, in the patient's interests, Amy called the trauma center to make sure this had been done prior to his discharge.

Taking call in a frontier practice involves the *ethics of availability.* Pam stated that she had a response time of 20 minutes, so she ensured she stayed in a location that made this timeframe possible. Bob talked about staying up all night (being available) with a myocardial infarction (MI) patient at his clinic, while Jim stated that he was always cognizant of his 15-minute response time when he was on call.

The ethics of availability extends to the concept of access to care or *distributive justice.* Bob implies that the discontinuation of 24/7 medical service in his community was an unethical decision, based on finances and not service. Pam clearly felt it was unethical to close clinics in communities that had no other access to health care services and shunt the money to larger communities that had many health care options. Pam also thought it was unethical not to have local mental health services available for the little girl who had been raped.

Participants also provided evidence to support the ethics of *stewardship*. NPs were cognizant of the strain some patient situations placed on resources in their community. They were also aware of this concept in an economic context when discussing the expense of treating cases in an emergency room that could have been managed in their clinics for significantly less money.

Professional ethics are involved in protecting confidentiality in frontier communities. The first awareness of this comes with the effort the participants made to protect the identity of their communities and, hence, the privacy of their patients. The theme *there's an art to it* refers to both the art and ethics of frontier NP practice. In many situations these are related. When faced with patients who would discuss private matters in public places, confidentiality may be breached. Preventing this breach of ethics without offending people is both an ethical decision and an artful skill developed by frontier NPs.

Out on a limb describes how frontier NPs can feel when faced with difficult situations. Deciding when to stitch a face or sew up a finger is an art which is developed by getting a feel for both the situation and the people involved. Giving people the news, deciding when and where to tell a patient that he or she has a terminal diagnosis, involves the art of nursing. Although all nurses and NPs are faced with ethical situations, this book brings the contextual ethical nuances of frontier NP practice to light.

◼ PERSONAL CHALLENGES

This section presents evidence related to personal challenges faced by frontier NPs. Stress related to personal challenges may affect both the NP's professional and personal life. Retention of frontier NPs may hinge on the individual NP's ability to cope with the challenges that accompany practice in the frontier, including adapting to the frontier culture or *way of life*. This involves a lack of anonymity and a blurring of social roles. These challenges were echoed in the narratives. Specifically, challenges related to *being on call* or *on duty* were noted by the participants. These challenges make it difficult to maintain a work–life balance that is conducive to one's personal mental health and healthy interpersonal relationships.

Dual relationships within the community can be challenging as well. Finding a balance between the stress of having family and friends as patients and the comfort of "being there for them" may take time and experience. In Sharp's study (2010), some NPs were not able to manage this aspect of frontier NP practice and therefore separated themselves from the community.

Frequent call duties are also a personal/professional challenge. It was evident in both Bob's and Ann's narratives that maintaining enough providers to share call was a priority. Call was also a factor for Jim, although in his situation, call was spread evenly among five providers, which made it more "palatable." Lori noted that frontier NP practice was not always "rosy," and that the long hours and call responsibilities made frontier practice challenging. The participants in this study have found strategies to cope with these challenges. Successful utilization of techniques mentioned in the narratives, such as wearing scrubs while on duty, leads to retention of providers. This in turn improves the health outcomes of frontier communities through access to local health care.

■ THEORETICAL CONSTRUCTS

In addition to concepts and narrative themes, there are theoretical constructs woven throughout the narratives. A construct is a highly abstract concept that cannot be measured or observed (Chinn & Kramer, 1999, p. 56). Constructs may have multiple meanings; their meaning can only be determined in the context in which they are used, in this case frontier NP practice. The theoretical constructs in the model are characteristic of the *environment* of frontier NP practice; they represent the geo-socio-psychological environment of frontier NP practice.

Two assumptions related to theoretical constructs were made for this book. First, the theoretical constructs evidenced in the narratives exist on a continuum. For example, the construct *independence* exists on a continuum from slightly independent to highly independent. Second, individual thematic constructs may be related to other constructs. For the purposes of this book this relationship will be expressed by a forward slash (/). Four theoretical constructs emerged from the narratives: independence, fear, intimacy, and isolation.

Independence/Fear

Independence is a word used repeatedly throughout the narratives. The need for independence was the motivating factor that sent both Bob and Amy into the frontier. An independent practice was implied in all the participant stories. Even Jim, who worked in a group practice, worked alone when he was on call. He described patient situations when he was handling ER emergencies independently.

Fear was explicitly mentioned by Bob when he used the word "scary" to describe an obstetrical emergency. Ann also stated that potential NP candidates were "frightened immediately" when they learned what the job expectations were. Fear was implicit in Ann's and Amy's stories involving emergency patient situations. In most of the narratives, fear can be attributed to the lack of professional support during emergent patient situations.

The participants' experiences indicate a relationship between the constructs of independence and fear. The more independent the practice, the more likely you will be presented with situations that are scary. Embedded in the construct of fear is the feeling of being out on a limb, a theme that emerged from Ann's and Lori's stories. It is the ability to overcome fear and act, or, as Amy states, "to make a decision" that leads to effective frontier practice.

Intimacy/Isolation

Intimacy and isolation may be considered constructs on opposite poles of the same continuum. Intimacy implies closeness or connectedness, whereas isolation implies aloneness, separateness, or nothingness. Isolation may be explicit, such as when used in the geographic sense, or implicit, when used in the psychosocial sense.

Intimacy is a theme woven through many of the stories. Bob states, "You get to know these people on a very intimate level," and Jim was surprised at how intimate you get with somebody else's life. Sue discusses the closeness that is a part of rural culture, the closeness which allows her to "cry with her patients." Pam talks about how nice and helpful rural folks are to strangers. A sense of closeness or connectedness is implied in the theme *reciprocity of care*, such as when Pam finds a Thanksgiving feast in her motel room or when Ann is offered the use of restrooms during home visits.

Isolation is also a theme woven through many of the narratives. For example, a long transport distance to reach a higher level of medical care was mentioned by all the participants. This supports the concept of the geographic isolation of frontier communities. Isolation is also one of the criteria for federal designation of frontier communities. The theme *flying solo*, from Bob's narrative, speaks directly to being on one's own, or alone. Bob also talks about being kept socially aloof at community events. Ann talks about the lack of other health care professionals in her community, Sue talks about combating professional isolation by precepting NP students, and Amy discusses handling emergency situations without backup. Pam talks about driving through isolated areas, traveling to and from frontier clinics.

Intimacy and isolation are related concepts embedded in the narratives. Participant stories indicate that the intimacy they experience with their patients may be partially rooted in geographic isolation. Therefore, intimacy may be the trade-off or benefit derived from isolation.

■ CONCLUSION

An analysis of the narratives revealed many interrelated concepts. Themes that emerged from the narratives exemplified some of these concepts. Both the themes and concepts represent different types of knowledge that frontier NPs use reciprocally to provide care for their patients and support their communities. This knowledge supports a model for effective frontier NP practice, a model that will be introduced in Chapter 12.

■ QUESTIONS FOR DISCUSSION

- The analysis of narrative evidence is partially accomplished through interpretation of meanings. Are there any additional concepts or themes that reveal themselves to you?
- Historically, how have nurses used political knowledge and influence to impact practice?
- Think of a recent patient situation that you managed. What *ways of knowing* or types of knowledge did you utilize?

REFERENCES

Carper, B. (1978). Fundamental patterns of knowing in nursing. *Advances in Nursing Science, 1*(1), 13–23.

Chinn, P. L., & Kramer, M. K. (1999). *Theory and nursing: Integrated knowledge development* (5th ed.). St. Louis, MO: Mosby.

Dewey, J. (1969–1991). The early works, the middle works, the later works. In J. Boydston (Ed.), *The collected works of John Dewey*. Carbondale: Southern Illinois University Press.

Gadow, S. (1995). Narrative and exploration: Toward a poetics of knowledge in nursing. *Nursing Inquiry, 2*, 211–214.

Lausten, G. (2013). What do nurse practitioners do? Analysis of a skills survey of nurse practitioners. *Journal of the American Association of Nurse Practitioners, 25*, 32–41.

Long, K., & Weinert, C. (1989). Rural nursing: Developing the theory base. *Scholarly Inquiry for Nursing Practice: An International Journal, 3*, 113–127.

Medina, M., & Castillo, P. (2006). Nursing education as a reflective practice. *Texto & Contexto Enfermagen, 15*(2), 303–311.

Nairn, S. (2004). Emergency care and narrative knowledge. *Journal of Advanced Nursing, 48*(1), 59–67.

Sharp, D. (2010). *Factors related to the recruitment and retention of nurse practitioners in rural areas* (Doctoral dissertation). Available from ProQuest Dissertation database. Retrieved from https://search.proquest.com/docview/613695577?accountid=40810

White, J. (1995). Patterns of knowing: Review, critique, and update. *Advances in Nursing Science, 17*(4), 73–86.

12

A Conceptual Model for Frontier Nursing Practice

The purpose of this book is to explicate concepts related to frontier nurse practitioner (NP) practice and utilize those concepts to develop a conceptual model for frontier NP practice. The purpose of a conceptual model is to guide practice by bringing the characteristics of a relatively unknown phenomenon, such as frontier NP practice, to light (Risjord, 2010, p. 173). This chapter begins with a review of concepts related to nursing models in general and then applies these concepts to the conceptual model developed in this book.

■ NURSING MODELS

Conceptual models provide a way of thinking about a phenomenon, a mental picture of how that phenomenon is put together and works (Rogers, 1973). When one thinks about frontier practice, certain ideas and notions come to mind. These ideas or notions become concepts that can be identified and defined. Furthermore, some of the concepts may be related to each other. These relationships are then clarified in relational statements indicating how the relationship informs the phenomenon in question. It is the relational statements that provide the foundation for a nursing model.

Nursing models are prescriptive, a guide for nursing action or intervention (Risjord, 2010, p. 180). Models for nursing guide practice in a manner that incorporates the ethics, values, and goals of nursing. This guidance may be related to practice, administration, research, or education. To take responsible action, one must consider all the ramifications and nuances of that action. This involves choices that may have ethical implications.

TABLE 12.1   Nurse of the Future: Metaparadigm Constructs

Person:	Environment:
The recipient of nursing care or services; persons may be individuals, families, groups, communities, or populations (AACN, 1998, p. 2, as cited in Massachusetts Department of Higher Education, 2010, p. 7)	The atmosphere, milieu, or conditions in which an individual lives, works, or plays (ANA, 2004, p. 47, as cited in Massachusetts Department of Higher Education, 2010, p. 7)
Health:	**Nursing:**
An experience that is often expressed in terms of wellness and illness, and may occur in the presence or absence of disease or injury (ANA, 2004, p. 5, as cited in Massachusetts Department of Higher Education, 2010, p. 8)	The protection, promotion, and optimization of health and abilities, prevention of illness and injury, alleviation of suffering through the diagnosis and treatment of human response, and advocacy in the care of individuals, families, groups, communities, and populations (ANA, 2001, p. 5, as cited in Massachusetts Department of Higher Education, 2010, p. 8)

AACN, American Association of Critical-Care Nurses; ANA, American Nurses Association.

Source: Masters (2013, p. 77).

Nursing models are concerned with aspects of practice that are related to nursing's sphere of influence or *metaparadigm*. Nursing's metaparadigm includes the person, health, nursing, and the environment. These four metaparadigm constructs are very broad and have multiple definitions. Therefore, specific nursing models have different definitions of the constructs depending upon the nature of the model (Fawcett, 1992). The model in this book utilizes the metaparadigm definitions outlined in Table 12.1. These definitions were chosen to represent areas of core competencies for the Nurse of the Future (NOF) project (Massachusetts Department of Higher Education, 2010, as cited in Masters, 2013).

These construct definitions take into account both the broad scope of practice and the wide area of influence that frontier NPs have. For example, the nursing outcomes in the conceptual model for frontier NP practice are related to both individuals and the community. This is congruent with the NOF definition of person. In addition, the NOF definition of environment is wide enough to encompass both the physical and the psychosocial environment of frontier NP practice. Also, the NOF definition of health is congruent with the concept of health in the frontier, one that focuses on the ability to work and be productive rather than on the absence of disease. Furthermore, the NOF definition of nursing takes into account advocacy for individuals or groups, an intervention that was clearly described in the narratives.

The frame of reference for the model developed in this book is frontier NP practice, a specialized type of advanced practice nursing. Different frames of reference allow models to function as guidelines for specific areas of nursing specialization (Rogers, 1973). As noted in Chapter 1, frontier NPs practice in the borderlands between nursing and medicine (Boyd, 2000; Hanson & Hamric, 2003). However, NPs approach their practice with a nursing mindset and are guided by the principles and values of the nursing profession. Therefore, the model for NP practice prescribes a distinct type of practice, one that is rooted in nursing (Ruel & Motyka, 2009).

▪ RELATIONAL STATEMENTS

As previously noted, conceptual models illustrate how concepts are interrelated. These relationships are clarified through the use of relational statements. In the model for frontier NP practice, these statements include:

- Frontier NPs practice independently; they manage chronic and emergent patient problems without backup

- Emergency services are lacking in the frontier; frontier NPs manage emergency and trauma situations

- Frontier NPs may practice solo; they utilize triage skills to manage multiple patient situations simultaneously

- Frontier NPs experience role diffusion; frontier practice requires a broad skillset

- Frontier NPs practice in professional isolation; they build interdisciplinary teams to enhance patient care

- Frontier NPs practice in environments with limited educational resources; they continually seek learning opportunities

- Frontier NPs practice in environments with limited resources; they use innovative strategies to provide patient care

- Mental health services are lacking in the frontier; frontier NPs require knowledge regarding the diagnosis and treatment of mental health problems

- Public health is lacking in the frontier; frontier NPs require knowledge regarding communicable and emerging diseases

- Frontier communities are culturally diverse; frontier NPs are culturally sensitive and possess knowledge that is specific to the setting

- Political forces impact frontier health care; frontier NPs use knowledge of federal policies and programs to stabilize local health care access

- State and federal policies change over time, so frontier clinics may close or merge with larger organizations; frontier NPs advocate for access to local health care

- Frontier NPs face a wide variety of ethical dilemmas; they utilize the concepts of patient autonomy, confidentiality, duty, stewardship, and distributive justice to navigate through patient situations that require ethical comportment

- Social capital is lacking in the frontier; NPs add to the social capital in their communities through leadership roles and personal commitment

These statements include interventions that require four types of knowledge, as discussed in Chapter 11: (a) frontier skills and competencies, (b) contextual knowledge, (c) political knowledge, and (d) art and ethics.

■ THE MODEL

Models are developed to guide nursing action toward a specified outcome or outcomes. In the model for frontier NP practice (see Figure 12.1), these outcomes include (a) stable access to local health care, (b) less reliance on hospital emergency departments for care, (c) an integrated approach to emergent patient situations, and (d) increased social capital.

These outcomes are the result of frontier NP praxis. Praxis constitutes nursing as a human caring practice and occurs when scientific competence, therapeutic use of self, moral–ethical comportment, and transformative

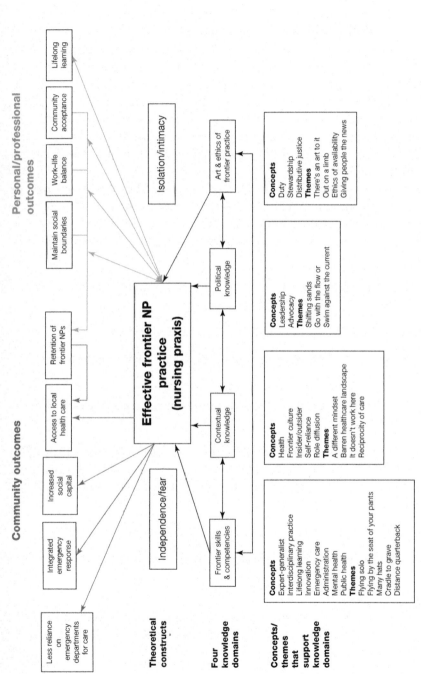

FIGURE 12.1 Conceptual model for frontier NP practice.
NP, nurse practitioner.

art/acts occur in synchrony (Chinn & Kramer, 1999, p. 256). In the model, praxis is conceptualized as effective frontier NP practice. It is considered effective because all participants in this book demonstrated effectiveness, not only in practice, but also in leadership and program administration.

Effective frontier NP practice is at the center of the model (see Figure 12.1). This practice is supported by four types of knowledge, as indicated by one-directional arrows. The arrows between the types of knowledge are bidirectional, indicating reciprocal relationships between them. Each type of knowledge is supported by concepts and themes from the narratives.

Effective frontier NP practice leads to enhanced provision of frontier health care. One-directional arrows from practice to community outcomes indicate this relationship. The relationship between effective frontier NP practice and community outcomes may be stated in the form of propositional statements, such as:

- Effective frontier NP practice leads to an integrated response to emergent patient situations.

- Effective NP practice stabilizes local health care.

- Effective NP practice increases the social capital in frontier communities.

- Effective NP practice reduces avoidable emergency department visits.

The model also includes personal/professional outcomes. The relationships between effective frontier NP practice and these outcomes are symbolized with bidirectional arrows. The assumptions underlying these relationships are:

- A healthy work–life balance leads to effective NP practice.

- An effective NP maintains appropriate social boundaries.

- Community acceptance enhances frontier NP practice.

- Frontier NPs who successfully manage the personal and professional challenges of frontier practice are more likely to stay in the frontier.

- The maintenance of a current knowledge base leads to effective NP practice.

A reciprocal relationship between personal/professional outcomes and community outcomes was not demonstrated in the narratives. However, NPs who successfully manage the personal challenges of frontier practice are more likely to be retained in those settings. Therefore, there is a one-directional relationship between personal outcomes and community outcomes.

The theoretical constructs of independence/fear and isolation/intimacy are in the center of the model. The constructs of independence/fear are relational constructs that emerged from stories involving clinical practice; therefore, they are placed above *competencies* and *contextual knowledge*. The constructs of isolation/fear are relational constructs that emerged from stories involving interpersonal relationships; therefore, they are situated above the *art and ethics* of frontier practice.

■ CONCLUSION

Concepts are ideas or notions that are specific to a certain phenomenon. Concepts may be related to one another. When these relationships bridge the gap between abstract notions and practical wisdom, they act as a guide for nursing practice. Relational statements form the basis for symbolic models that can be depicted visually as diagrams. The diagram of the model resulting from the participant interviews is depicted in Figure 12.1. Models that include measurable outcomes can be tested through research. Linking nursing interventions to positive patient or community outcomes informs nursing science. The community outcomes in this model can be tested using a variety of research designs.

The authority for the model lies in nursing's metaparadigm, the components of which are evident in the model: person, health, environment, and nursing. The validity for the model lies within the narratives of NPs who live the experience of frontier practice. The participants were recruited from five different western states and represent a variety of frontier health care models. This participant criterion enhances the transferability of the model to other frontier practice settings.

The model is a guide for frontier NP practice. It is built on the knowledge of NPs who have demonstrated nursing praxis in their communities. The model is also an example of practice informing theory regarding the salient features of frontier nursing practice.

The theory underlying the research for the model is pragmatism. Therefore, the model is a pragmatic guide for frontier NP practice because it is based on concepts that are important to those who practice there.

The model also informs nurse educators regarding the distinct nature of frontier NP practice and the specific educational preparation and prerequisite experience required for effective frontier practice.

▪ QUESTIONS FOR DISCUSSION

- Have you ever utilized a nursing model in practice?
- Can you remember a nursing situation where your interventions may have been enhanced through the use of a nursing model?
- Think of a research question that might stem from this model. How might you design a study to answer your question?

REFERENCES

Boyd, L. (2000). Advanced practice nursing today. *RN, 63*(9), 57–62.

Chinn, P. L., & Kramer, M. K. (1999). *Theory and nursing: Integrated knowledge development* (5th ed.). St. Louis, MO: Mosby.

Fawcett, J. (1991). Conceptual models and nursing practice: The reciprocal relationship. *Journal of Advanced Nursing, 17*, 224–228.

Hanson, C. M., & Hamric, A. B. (2003). Reflections on the continuing evolution of advanced practice nursing. *Nursing Outlook, 51*, 203–211.

Masters, K. (2013). *Role development in professional nursing practice* (3rd ed.). Burlington, MA: Jones & Bartlett.

Risjord, M. (2010). *Nursing knowledge: Science, practice, and philosophy.* Chichester, West Sussex, UK: Wiley-Blackwell.

Rogers, C. G. (1973). Conceptual models as guides to clinical nursing specialization. *Journal of Nursing Education, 12*(4), 2–6.

Ruel, J., & Motyka, C. (2009). Advanced practice nursing: A principle-based concept analysis. *Journal of the American Academy of Nurse Practitioners, 21*, 384–392.

13

Recommendations and Conclusions

Part I of this book paints a picture of life in the frontier for both frontier dwellers and frontier health care providers. This picture includes challenges regarding the provision of health care in the frontier. Part II provides examples of how frontier communities and nurse practitioners (NPs) are meeting these challenges and, in some cases, overcoming them. These challenges include workforce, emergency medical services (EMS), and educational issues. The conceptual model for frontier NP practice provides guidelines, or recommendations, in each of these areas. This chapter begins with a review of these guidelines.

■ NURSING EDUCATION

There are two recommendations from the Institute of Medicine's report on the future of nursing that have implications for frontier NP education (Institute of Medicine (US), Committee on the Robert Wood Johnson Foundation Initiative on the Future of Nursing, 2011). First, identify the features of online, simulation, and tele-health nursing education that most cost-effectively expand nursing education capacity. Second, identify and test new and existing models of education to support nurses' engagement in team-based, patient-centered care to diverse populations, across the life span, in a range of settings.

To prepare nurses to work in the frontier setting, the challenge is twofold. First, identify and recruit candidates who are likely to practice in the frontier. This includes developing online and hybrid programs that allow students who live in frontier communities to receive the bulk of their education while staying in these communities. The second challenge is to develop educational programs that prepare NPs for the distinct type of practice conceptualized in the model. Based on the narrative evidence underlying the model, the following recommendations are presented:

- Frontier NPs provide primary and emergency care to patients of all ages. Therefore, to practice in frontier communities, NPs must be prepared as family NPs. This licensure allows the broadest scope of practice.

- Mental health services are severely lacking in frontier communities. Frontier NPs need the knowledge required to treat mental health patients safely and effectively.

- Trauma care is inevitable in the frontier. NP programs may not be accredited to provide training in this area. Therefore, NP programs should educate students regarding this aspect of frontier practice and provide suggestions for where NPs can receive this preparation.

- Professional isolation is common in the frontier. Preparing students to use both formal and informal resources is paramount to reduce the effects of this isolation.

- Most frontier NPs have on-call obligations that can be challenging both professionally and personally. NPs who wish to practice in the frontier require strong mentorship from a provider who has developed the means to cope with these challenges.

- NPs who wish to practice in the frontier should be educated on the various federal and state programs that affect frontier NP practice and the delivery of frontier health care.

- Ethical content should include the ethics of availability and ethical comportment when dealing with life-and-death situations in the frontier. Leadership and advocacy in frontier settings are issues that can be discussed and promoted within an ethical framework.

Some participants in this book were prepared in NP programs whose mission was to educate NPs for rural practice. None of the participants received *any* specialized education regarding rural or frontier issues. Course content in rural NP education tracts should support an expert-generalist skillset; courses could provide content regarding several issues related to rural/frontier health care:

- Rural/frontier demographics

- Rural/frontier culture

- Health status/disparities

- Rural/frontier economies

- Rural/frontier health issues, specifically related to extractive industries and agriculture

- Adequacy or availability of rural/frontier public health

- Rural/frontier health care delivery models

- Effect of the Affordable Care Act (ACA), specifically regarding rural accountable care organizations and value-based payment systems

- Research on rural and frontier nursing

Although this is not an exhaustive list, it recognizes the distinctive nature of frontier nursing. Depending upon the local industries, programs could also provide intensive experiences to prepare students for the most common industrial-related injuries in their geographic setting.

■ RESEARCH

The model provides a framework for research involving various aspects of frontier health care delivery. The outcome, *less reliance on emergency departments for care*, could be determined by chart audits and a review of after-hour cases seen by the NP. For example, the electronic medical record system tracts both the time of day a patient was seen and the type of visit. A researcher could audit the after-hour visits to determine the number of patients who avoided emergency department visits due to the availability of local care. If it could be proven that significant health care dollars were saved, some of those funds might be utilized to offset the cost of paying an on-call provider.

Ann noted that often patient emergencies could be managed at her clinic without extended transport times and the increased cost of an acute care emergency room. The outcome, *integrated emergency response*, might involve an audit of run reviews to determine how quickly emergency patients received initial care, by whom (what skill level), and the length of transport time to definitive care. This time might include transport time to a trauma center, local hospital, or a rural clinic. An investigation of this type might also determine what percentage of time a community was left without the available ambulance services, a phenomenon that occurs in the event of long transport times. Results could lead to expanded or new agreements for mutual coverage by other agencies.

Interventional studies are also an option. For example, providing relevant and convenient continuing education on topics such as medical treatment for depression could improve management of patients in frontier areas. The effectiveness of the intervention could be demonstrated through the use of patient pre- and postintervention depression scores.

Organizations interested in frontier workforce retention could survey frontier providers regarding their intent to stay in frontier practice. For those providers who indicate a desire to leave, the model could provide a framework to determine what causal factors were included in their decision-making process. Through ameliorating reversible factors, some practitioners could potentially decide to stay in frontier practice. For example, efforts to bring in a relief provider for a few days a month might relieve enough stress to allow a provider to stay in the community.

■ HEALTH CARE POLICY

Frontier Health Care Workforce

Chapter 2 presented evidence that recruitment and retention of frontier providers are problematic. Chapter 3 presented research regarding recruitment schemes and retention theories. The literature suggests that being close to family or having been raised in a rural area enhanced recruitment and retention of frontier providers. In particular, Sharp (2010) listed proximity to family as a likely reason for nurses to stay in rural/frontier areas.

There are also recruitment strategies, such as loan repayment models, mentioned in the review. The literature is also rife with information regarding rural rotations and immersion experiences for nursing and medical students. However, participants in this book came to the frontier for the following reasons:

- A desire for autonomy and independence

- To provide a service in communities where they were raised (grow your own)

- To be near family

- For the lifestyle

There may be personality characteristics that are predictive of successful rural or frontier NP practice. In Colledge's (2000) study of hardiness as a predictor of NPs in rural practice, she found that hardiness did not predict success in rural areas. However, Colledge did find that nurses who scored higher on the challenge subscale were more likely to practice effectively in rural/frontier areas. Challenge may be related to the constructs of autonomy and independence, reasons cited by participants as a motivation to enter frontier NP practice. Therefore, nursing schools may want to explore personality traits when considering applicants for rural/frontier tracts.

National Health Service Corp (NHSC) loan repayment commitments are offered for 2-year terms of service. Although this commitment exposes NPs to the frontier/rural practice environment, it does little to encourage retention. The participants in this book had experience with four such NHSC loan repayment recipients. None of the four stayed past their 2-year commitment. Family reasons were most commonly cited as reasons for leaving. However, this should not be taken to indicate that the program has no merit. Although the NHSC loan repayment program did not provide long-term coverage for the frontier clinics involved in this study, it did provide short-term coverage solutions and respite for the NPs who worked with them. It also provided recipients experiences in patient situations not likely to be found elsewhere.

An evidence-based solution to this problem would seem to be the grow-your-own model. A recent study demonstrated that all frontier counties in the study's data set had at least one RN (Jakobs, 2014). RNs living in frontier communities who desire to further their education should be encouraged and supported to do so. These RNs could be supported by educational grants and loan repayment programs such as the NHSC. Educational opportunities that combine distance education with local preceptorships would support this concept. Programs such as the RN to Doctor of Nursing Practice (DNP) could fast-track these students.

Emergency Services

The narrative evidence in this book paints the picture of a very fragile and fragmented frontier EMS system. This finding supports a previous study of EMS in rural areas of this country. That study indicated that frontier EMS systems have difficulty staffing and recruiting enough volunteers to provide timely patient transport to emergency or trauma departments (Knott, 2003).

The availability of air transport does not entirely mitigate these issues. The participants in this book stated that there was a minimum of 35 minutes to an hour for air transport to reach the scene of the emergency or to a safe landing zone. Air transport may also be hampered by poor weather conditions. Additionally, geographic conditions may necessitate the availability of ambulance services to transport patients to a safe landing zone.

Transport times may also be lengthening due to the increase in rural hospital closures, resulting in longer transport times from frontier communities to the nearest emergency department. The National Advisory Committee on Rural Health and Human Services recently published a policy brief to address the loss of rural emergency departments (2016). The committee proposes several alternative models to preserve access to emergency care. One option, or alternative model, was proposed for communities that are too small to support a 24-hour emergency department; it is consistent with some characteristics of the participant models in this book. This option includes the creation of a primary care clinic that would be open 8 to 12 hours a day with an adjacent ambulance service operating 24/7, creating a clinic by day, and a stabilize-and-transfer model by night. Medicare could reimburse primary care visits and ambulance transports, but also provide a fixed supplemental amount to support the capital costs of operating a primary care practice, the standby costs of the ambulance service, and costs of uncompensated care. The committee recommendations support the notion that NPs and their respective frontier clinics should be considered part of the prehospital system in their local communities or regions.

The experiences of participants in this study indicate poor formal integration with local EMS systems. This is unfortunate for a variety of reasons. First, in communities where only basic life support (BLS) services are available, the local NP is most likely the highest trained health care provider available and may represent the only advanced care life support within a 50- to 150-mile radius. Second, it has been the experience of several participants in this inquiry that trauma and cardiac patients present themselves directly to clinics—clinics that do not carry life-saving medications. Lastly, in frontier areas, the *golden hour* can be lost through the amount of time it takes to get volunteer EMS personnel to the scene.

NPs can mitigate at least part of this lost time by stabilizing trauma and cardiac patients prior to transport.

Evidence in this book illustrates that NPs are providing trauma and emergency medical care in frontier clinics across the country. Evidence in the literature also illustrates that trauma and cardiac patients are dying in frontier areas due to a lack of timely, integrated care. The model offers the following guidelines related to the integration of life saving EMS in frontier communities:

- NPs should be recognized and integrated into the EMS system

- 24/7 on-call coverage by a provider who holds advanced cardiac life support (ACLS) certification

- ACLS medications on the ambulance and in the clinic

- An alternative base station status for the EMS-integrated frontier clinics; this would allow patients to be transported to the clinic, if necessary, and be stabilized prior to further transport

- Reliable communication systems between volunteers, clinic, and tertiary hospital

- Available local x-ray services

- Volunteer EMS personnel should be given an alternative scope of practice that allows for insertion of IVs and the provision of IV fluids, epinephrine, and albuterol under specific standardized protocols or while under personal or radio supervision by the NP

As noted in Chapter 1, most frontier communities are surrounded by public lands. This has a negative effect on the ability to fund EMS systems in these frontier areas. The federal government has recognized this, and in years past has provided frontier counties with PILT (payment in lieu of taxes) funds to support services in these counties. These PILT funds are primarily utilized to fund firefighting, police protection, construction of public schools and roads, and search-and-rescue operations; however, this funding has decreased over recent years (U.S. Department of the Interior, n.d.).

The narratives also indicate a shift in health care funding. This shift appears to be away from communities that experience spatial health care inequity and toward population centers. Thus, frontier communities may interpret this as federal abandonment of frontier counties in this country, counties where most of the land is held in public trust. The funding and staffing of integrated frontier health care models takes creativity, tenacity, and federal support. It is important that this occurs, because the reality of the frontier EMS system is that you may dial 911 and no one comes to help you.

■ RECOMMENDATIONS FOR FURTHER RESEARCH

There is a paucity of research regarding frontier NP practice and frontier health care in general. Recommendations for further research are based on the narrative evidence presented in this book. Embedded in the recommendations for further research is the notion that NPs are inexplicitly involved with frontier health care. The participants in this book were all older than 50 and worried about their replacement. This is a valid concern and one that is worth further exploration.

Further research into the distribution of both rural and frontier NPs is warranted, as the last survey of NPs was conducted in 2000. To adequately conduct frontier nursing research, an updated survey of rural NP distribution should be conducted using established rural and frontier criteria. Some state boards of nursing report the distribution of advanced practice registered nurses (APRNs) within their state, but do not list the specific category of APRN, such as NP. The same situation exists when conducting a zip-code search using national provider identifier (NPI) numbers. The NPI does not distinguish an NP from an APRN. With the expansion of electronic billing and electronic medical records, researchers may have the opportunity to develop an accurate method to determine frontier NP distribution.

Further exploration into the economic impact that frontier clinics have on their community is warranted. Funding priorities are shifting to both population-based models and evidence-based models. Further studies to determine the amount of money and valuable emergency department resources saved when frontier patients are treated locally would support subsidizing 24/7 medical coverage in frontier communities.

The diversity of clinics and settings in this book illustrate the point that *it is not feasible* to have a one-size-fits-all model for the delivery of frontier health care. This statement is supported by the National Advisory Committee on Rural Health and Human Services, which states that no single model will fit all rural/frontier communities (2016, p. 8). Further research to determine which model best fits with the needs of specific communities would be beneficial.

CONCLUSION

The model in this book provides a guide for frontier NP practice from an emic, or insider, perspective. The participant narratives represent the reality, or ontology, of frontier NP practice. It is the assumption of this book that frontier NP practice is distinct from practice in other settings, a distinctive practice that few are aware of. The conceptual model for frontier NP practice, which resulted from participant narratives, is a guideline for practice, education, research, and policy into this distinct practice.

Frontier NPs provide a vital link in the overall scheme of frontier health care in the United States. Furthermore, NPs must have specific knowledge to practice effectively in frontier settings. To withstand the shifting sands of federal and state policy, frontier NPs must be informed and united in their cause: the cause of providing access to primary and emergency health care in frontier settings. The goal of this book is to give voice to NPs who are working in remote, isolated areas of the country. It is vital to the future of frontier health care that this chorus of voices be heard.

QUESTIONS FOR DISCUSSION

- What would be an ideal model to prepare NPs for frontier practice?
- What further recommendations could be made based on the participant narratives?
- Some people may suggest that frontier communities fund their own EMS system. Do you believe this is plausible? Do you believe this is ethical?

REFERENCES

Colledge, P. (2000). *Hardiness as a predictor of nurse practitioners in rural practice* (Doctoral dissertation). Available from ProQuest Dissertation database. Retrieved from https://search.proquest.com/docview /304627597?accountid=40810

Institute of Medicine (US), Committee on the Robert Wood Johnson Foundation Initiative on the Future of Nursing. (2011). *The future of nursing:*

Leading change, advancing health. Washington, DC: National Academies Press.

Jakobs, L. (2014, July). *APRNs and the population's health in frontier communities.* Poster presentation at the International Rural Health and Rural Nursing Research Conference, Bozeman, MT.

Knott, A. (2003). Emergency medical services in rural areas: The supporting role of state EMS agencies. *The Journal of Rural Health, 19*(4), 492–496. doi:10.1111/j.1748-0361.2003.tb00587.x

National Advisory Committee on Rural Health and Human Services. (2016, July). *Alternative models to preserving access to emergency care* (Policy brief). Retrieved from http://www.hrsa.gov/advisorycommittees/rural/publications/alternatemodel.pdf

Sharp, D. (2010). *Factors related to the recruitment and retention of nurse practitioners in rural areas* (Doctoral dissertation). Available from ProQuest Dissertation database. Retrieved from https://search.proquest.com/docview/613695577?accountid=40810

U.S. Department of the Interior. (n.d.). Payments in lieu of taxes. Retrieved from www.doi.gov/pilt/index.cfm

APPENDIX

Useful Websites

Amber Waves
https://www.ers.usda.gov/amber-waves.aspx

Center for Rural Health, North Dakota
https://ruralhealth.und.edu

National Center for Frontier Communities
http://frontierus.org

North Carolina Rural Health Research and Policy Analysis Center
https://www.ruralhealthresearch.org/centers/northcarolina

Rural Health Information Hub
https://www.ruralhealthinfo.org/topics

South Carolina Rural Research Center
http://rhr.sph.sc.edu

The Daily Yonder
http://www.dailyyonder.com

Index